*Baba's Kitchen Medicines*

MICHAEL MUCZ

# Baba's Kitchen Medicines

FOLK REMEDIES

OF UKRAINIAN SETTLERS

IN WESTERN CANADA

The University of Alberta Press

Published by
The University of Alberta Press
Ring House 2
Edmonton, Alberta, Canada T6G 2E1
www.uap.ualberta.ca

Library and Archives Canada Cataloguing in Publication

Mucz, Michael, 1947-
    Baba's kitchen medicines : folk remedies of Ukrainian
settlers in Western Canada / Michael Mucz.

Includes bibliographical references and index.
ISBN 978-0-88864-514-2

    1. Ukrainian Canadians--Medicine--Prairie Provinces.
2. Ukrainians--Medicine--Prairie Provinces.  3. Traditional
medicine--Prairie Provinces.  I. Title.

GR113.7.U57M89 2011      398'.353      C2010-908137-4

First edition, first printing, 2012.
Printed and bound in Canada by Houghton Boston Printers, Saskatoon, Saskatchewan.
Copyediting and Proofreading by Elizabeth Macfie and Svitlana Krys.
Maps by Wendy Johnson.
Indexing by Judy Dunlop.

The University of Alberta Press is committed to protecting our natural environment. As part of our
efforts, this book is printed on Enviro Paper: it contains 100% post-consumer recycled fibres and is
acid- and chlorine-free.

The University of Alberta Press gratefully acknowledges the support received for its publishing
program from The Canada Council for the Arts. The University of Alberta Press also gratefully
acknowledges the financial support of the Government of Canada through the Canada Book Fund
(CBF) and the Government of Alberta through the Alberta Multimedia Development Fund (AMDF)
for its publishing activities.

*To the memories of the Ukrainian pioneer men, women, and children who endured unimaginable challenges in order to make a better life for themselves and those that followed. May their faith, courage, and accomplishments be a source of inspiration and strength to all Canadians.*

# Disclaimer  ✍

The information contained in this book is presented solely for general educational purposes and represents historical documentation of the traditional folk medicine practices used by Ukrainian settlers in western Canada. These treatments were widely used on homesteads when doctors and hospitals were unavailable or difficult to access. The remedies and treatments are not presented as advice or prescription for self-treatment. No guarantee is made as to the accuracy, completeness, or safety of these home remedies or treatments. It is strongly recommended that you consult a physician for appropriate advice on any medical condition. The author and the University of Alberta Press accept no personal liability for inappropriate use of the information presented in this book.

Know your limits and recognize that good sense and health not only go together but are also life's greatest blessings. Make your personal health a valued and lifelong task.

# Contents   ♬

# Tables  🦎

# Maps  🐎

# Abbreviations 🖎

PAA Provincial Archives of Alberta

PAM Provincial Archives of Manitoba

# Acknowledgements   ✒

My sincerest appreciation goes out to all the women and men who so generously and patiently shared their personal—and at times painful—recollections. Even though I prodded and directed them with specific questions, they often took opportunities to expand and enliven their answers with the warmth of memories long held but rarely shared.

The staff of many Ukrainian seniors' centres, lodges, and nursing homes generously identified and solicited knowledgeable informants for me to work with. Without their help, my informant base would have been considerably reduced and the study's contents severely limited. Many individuals also shared names of relatives, friends, or acquaintances who proved to be invaluable sources of information. To all of you generous people, I am deeply indebted for the trust you showed in me and in this study.

Some individuals do, however, stand out as being critical to the direction and success of this project. Julie Hrapko, the former Curator of Botany at the Royal Alberta Museum (Edmonton), was instrumental in encouraging, directing, and supporting me in my undertaking of this study. Radomir Bilash, senior Ukrainian historian with Historic Sites Service, Alberta, and onsite historian for the Ukrainian Cultural Heritage Village Historical Site, provided numerous insights, encouragement, and access to his extensive research materials. My wife, Brenda, was unselfish in her willingness to do more than her share of looking after our household, including our infant twin sons, as I made long and time-consuming research trips to interview informants. Her support and many sacrifices allowed me the time and opportunity to fulfill my passion for this study. As well, my deepest gratitude goes to Michael Luski, former Acquisitions

Editor for the University of Alberta Press, for his encouragement, support, and guidance in seeing that my manuscript became worthy of publication. I am also deeply appreciative of the kindness and support I received from Mary Lou Roy and Alan Brownoff during the publication process. To the many others who have not been acknowledged directly but did contribute to this study, I also extend genuine thanks. Please know that any and all credit that this work may generate, I gratefully and readily share with you all.

The Government of Alberta provided extensive financial support for travel, accommodations, and supplies. The University of Alberta (Augustana Faculty) provided me with both research funds and two sabbatical leaves to research and synthesize this study.

Financial publication support was provided by the Canadian Foundation for Ukrainian Studies, in the form of a grant from its Scholarly Publications Support Program.

Last, but by no means least, I express deeply felt gratitude to my parents, Peter and Ann, who gave me my Ukrainian heritage, encouraged its growth within me, and provided me with the educational opportunities to ultimately rediscover it.

Thank you very much *(Ia vam duzhe diakuiu)*.

# Introduction  ✍

Our identity bears both hereditary and cultural lineages that shape who we are and how our lives have unfolded. This study provided me with the opportunity to connect with my own Ukrainian heritage and better understand its significant cultural impacts on the development of western Canada.

People strive to improve their lot in life, and if they are unable to reach that goal, then they try to provide that opportunity for their children. The Ukrainian settlers who immigrated to western Canada in the late 1800s and early 1900s embodied this spirit of a quest for a better life. Hardships, sacrifice, and uncertainty became daily challenges of life on frontier homesteads. The adversities they faced were more than offset by their deep religious faith and remarkable spirit of perseverance. The capacity of both young and old to work long and hard under demanding conditions became a significant survival attribute. The Ukrainian settlers not only overcame the wilderness challenges of their newly adopted country, but lived to prosper from the bountiful opportunities and abundant natural resources it provided.

As my elderly informants vividly recalled memories of those early days, there were numerous occasions when the tone of their voice noticeably weakened and quivered. For some, tears stained their face as they struggled to tell of the seemingly endless hardships and challenges of homestead life. Other recollections brought strength to their words and pride to their faces as they described their own family's, or subsequent generations', accomplishments. The trials, tribulations, and successes of the Ukrainian settlers are not isolated or unique in western Canadian history. Many other ethnic groups achieved similar results through similar efforts.

Even though the human capacity for forming and retaining memory deteriorates with age, early memories and experiences typically remain strong and clear. It was with these early recollections that my informants allowed me to "see" how their grandparents or parents survived the early settlement years on isolated homesteads.

Based on this diverse wealth of collected information, most of it recorded on audiotape, I intend to write a series of books on features of Ukrainian homestead life in western Canada. This book, on the use of home remedies by the early Ukrainian settlers, is but the first. It is my hope that this book will serve as an everlasting tribute, and a personal record of the accomplishments and legacy left behind by our Ukrainian pioneers. Their knowledge and practices provide us with a wealth of information to study, learn from, and possibly apply to our own lives.

Therefore it is their story, written with sweat and tears, and not mine. To them goes all recognition, praise, and gratitude for all that they were so willing to share. My own expressions of deep appreciation for what they had given me were most often met with the simple reply, "For what *(dlia choho)*?" This humble yet powerful response readily captures the unselfish generosity of the pioneer spirit.

My greatest regret is that I did not undertake this study a decade or so earlier, when many of the original settlers were still alive. I am nevertheless grateful that God gave me the opportunity to record vestiges of their memories that, unfortunately, are gradually fading and being lost as they and their offspring pass on. In sharing their knowledge with others, I live up to the promise that I made to all my informants. What they shared so freely and unconditionally with me would be similarly shared with others. The past is a rich and relatively untapped resource that has much to offer us in the present. I can only hope that this book is read in that spirit.


## ABOUT THE AUTHOR

I am a Ukrainian Canadian who came to Canada, as a child, after World War II under the designation of a displaced person (DP). Both of my parents were from the western Ukrainian region of Galicia, and they immigrated to Canada because my father's father and uncle were already here working on the railway. My early years were spent at a Ukrainian settlement site in East Selkirk, Manitoba, and my formative years were spent growing up in the ethnically diverse north end of Winnipeg.

My post-secondary education involved a BSc (Honours) in botany and zoology at the University of Manitoba, and a PhD in plant ecology at the University of Alberta. My one and only permanent job, teaching biology at the university level, began at Camrose Lutheran College, which later became Augustana University College and is now the Augustana Faculty of the University of Alberta. Teaching has provided me with thirty-five years of opportunity to learn and grow in an academic environment. This book is therefore a wonderful milestone in a most enjoyable professional career.

For a number of years, Julie Hrapko, a fellow Ukrainian Canadian, who at the time was the Curator of Botany at the Provincial Museum in Edmonton, had been encouraging ethnobotanical studies of major Albertan ethnic groups. Since I was fluent in Ukrainian, she encouraged me study this major group that had settled throughout western Canada, and extensively so in east central Alberta.

## STUDY METHODOLOGY

In 1992, with a sabbatical leave from the University, I initiated this ethnobotanical study of home remedies used by Ukrainian settlers in western Canada. I quickly realized that I was probably ten to fifteen years too late to access the original Ukrainian settlers (my informants' parents and grandparents). My main resources were therefore their immediate—and in some cases their later—descendants and relatives who still possessed clear memories of their homestead upbringing. These informants provided me with rich and diversified recollections of pioneer life in the early days of Ukrainian settlement, primarily in east central Alberta.

My initial approach in locating suitable informants was to contact and visit senior citizens' lodges and nursing homes in the cities, towns, and villages of east central Alberta (Map 1). The residents of these facilities became a major source of the information in this book. I also visited the local community seniors' centres and was able to identify additional informants who were still living on their own. The majority of informants were in Andrew, Camrose, Chipman, Edmonton, Holden, Innisfree, Lamont, Mundare, Smoky Lake, Two Hills, Vegreville, Willingdon, and surrounding areas. This was geographically

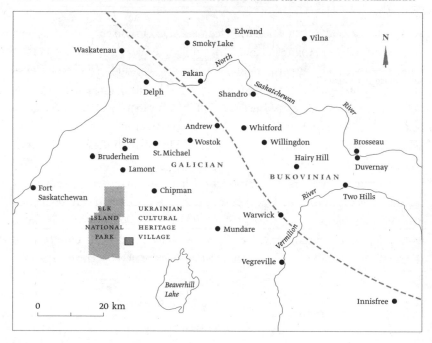

similar to the area Robert Klymasz studied for his 1992 publication *Svieto*, which dealt with celebratory rituals practised by Ukrainians in east central Alberta.

I formally interviewed and audiotaped almost 200 informants and contacted countless more in a less formal manner. Information (discussions, letters, etc.) from additional informants was also collected but not recorded. Each recorded interview, conducted in English or Ukrainian and taped with a cassette recorder, lasted one to two hours. The interview began with a summary of the informant's personal history and then focused on use of native or domestic plants in various personal, household, or homestead activities or practices (see Appendix I). My main goal was to understand traditional healing materials and practices used in the informant's family of origin, as well as in the adjacent Ukrainian settlement area. Each informant was asked to sign a waiver release form, permitting the use of the recorded material. All audiotapes will be deposited in the Provincial Archives of Alberta for other researchers to use.

TABLE 1    Profile of informants (total = 191) interviewed for this study

| Gender | |
|---|---|
| | Females: 133 (70%) |
| | Males: 58 (30%) |
| *Age* (average and range) | |
| | Females: 81 yrs. (age 51–97) |
| | Males: 81 yrs. (age 65–91) |
| *Family origins* | |
| | Galicia: 99 (52%) |
| | Bukovina: 63 (33%) |
| | Uncertain: 29 (15%) |
| *Religion* | |
| | Ukrainian (Greek) Catholic: 88 (46%) |
| | Ukrainian Greek Orthodox: 71 (37%) |
| | Russian Orthodox: 13 (7%) |
| | Roman Catholic: 12 (6%) |
| | Other: 7 (4%) |
| *Family size* (average number of children) | |
| | Family of origin: 7.1 |
| | Own family: 3.7 |

The informant profiles (Table 1) show that twice as many women as men were interviewed, but that their average age (81 years) was the same. The majority of their families of origin were from Galicia and most were of the Ukrainian Greek Catholic or Ukrainian Greek Orthodox faiths. The number of children that the informants had themselves was only about half of the number their parents had. This shows that during the homestead period, large families were the norm and children were an important source of farm labour.

Additional materials were gathered from a variety of available published resources: local community and family histories, as well as various books (see

Selected Readings) on subjects dealing with Ukrainian settlement in western Canada. Unpublished materials (notes, personal documents) were also used.

To better evaluate the various home remedies and treatments used, I calculated a treatment value (TV) factor, which allowed me to quantitatively identify the most widely used healing practices and materials. The TV factor took into consideration the number of informants (NI) reporting the use of the practice or materials and the number of different health conditions (HC) that these were used for. Use of the square root of NI ensured that the informant number factor, which naturally was the larger number, did not outweigh the importance of the number of conditions treated with the specific practice or material.

$$TV = HC \sqrt{NI}$$

The higher the TV value for any home remedy, the more important its use in traditional healing. It is primarily the number of users that is most influential in determining which of the remedies were of the greatest use in the settlement communities.


## TEXT FEATURES

Ukrainian words and phrases are presented using the Library of Congress system of transliteration (see Appendix V). These are presented in *italicized* type, within parentheses ( ), immediately after their equivalent English word(s). For example: in the Old Country *(u kraiu)*. These provide emphasis and effect to interview content and reflect the folk-like terminology common to rural people. I hope that readers familiar with the Ukrainian language will more readily recognize the term's significance and application in the stated context.

In descriptions of healing practices and materials used, all home remedies and treatments are grouped in three categories: Drinking, Eating, and Applying. The latter describes a non-consumptive method of treatment. I will *italicize* the major treatment method(s), identify the most commonly used material(s) in **bold text**, separate the variety of materials used in the same manner by means of a forward slash ( / ), and identify other materials used in a different manner by separating them with a bullet (·).

For example:

***Drinking:***
- *Infusion* of: **chamomile** flowers / red willow bark / wormwood.
- regular tea.

Throughout the book I provide personalized treatment stories for specific conditions. Each story is identified by its informant's initials and his or her hometown in Alberta. For example:

> *I knew a man who had gangrene on his foot and the doctor had suggested amputation. Someone told him that this was not necessary, because he could cure it himself by soaking the foot in warm wormwood solution for a few weeks. He did this and his leg healed up. All he was left with was a slight limp.*
> — E. K. / Edmonton

# ONE

# Immigration and Settlement

The first, and most significant, of three Ukrainian immigration waves to Canada consisted of 170,000 to 200,000 individuals, occurred between 1890 and 1914, and was in response to a federal government recruiting program in Eastern Europe. The government's objective was to establish western regional sovereignty through rapid development and settlement of Canada's western territories. Suitable individuals were sought out to immigrate and develop homesteads in the West's southern and central regions. Sir Clifford Sifton, Minister of the Interior and Immigration during the early period, stated, "I think that a stalwart peasant in a sheepskin coat, born on the soil, whose forefathers have been farmers for ten generations, with a stout wife and a half dozen children, is good quality." Ukrainian peasants, identified as "rooted" in the soil, possessed a strong and successful agricultural heritage and fit these requirements perfectly. They were well suited for such a colonization program and were vigorously recruited for this task. Canada also needed an extensive manual labour force for its forestry, mining, agriculture, and construction (railroad and urban) industries, and once again the Ukrainians were well suited to these needs, with their strong backs, willing arms, and admirable work ethic.

The majority of Ukrainian immigrants came from two provincial regions of the Austro-Hungarian Empire: Galicia (Halychyna) was an area of western Ukraine bordering eastern Poland, and Bukovina (Bukovyna) was an area of southwestern Ukraine bordering Romania (Map 2). The initial Ukrainian immigrants were officially identified on their documents as Ruthenians, Austrians, Russians, Galicians, or Bukovinians because of the continuously changing geopolitical borders of the regions from which they emigrated. Most of these early

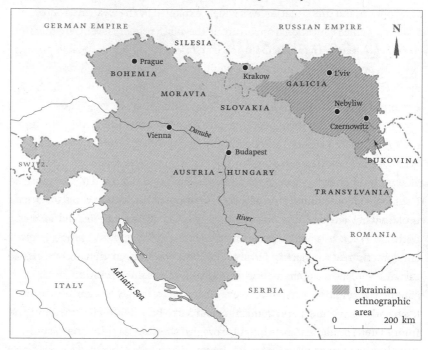

Ukrainian immigrants were rural, agrarian, land poor, and relatively uneducated. They had only recently, in the mid-1800s, been granted freedom from serfdom, and much of their agricultural and forested lands were occupied by extensive estates run by wealthy and oppressive lords *(pany)*. These wealthy landowners were more than satisfied to see the relatively landless peasants and their future generations kept in poverty, misery, and despair, which provided them with an extensive source of cheap manual labour.

Additional oppressive restrictions on the peasants were to be found in the compulsory three-year military service in the Austro-Hungarian army for all males when they reached the age of eighteen, significant regional political instability and tension, limited educational opportunities for their children, an economic inability to increase land holdings, and a lack of access to free wood for building materials and fuel. Extremely small homesteads, only two or three hectares in size, were typical for the common folk, and many families owned no land at all. In most cases, this meant that working on the large estates was the only survival option, and this situation was widely exploited by the wealthy landowners. Children, denied educational opportunities beyond a primary level, were therefore forced to enter the manual labour force at an early age. It was obvious that the fortunes of future generations were going to worsen rather than improve. Such bleak conditions and prospects made strong emigration incentives, which were enhanced by the Canadian government's appealing offers of "free" land.

Thousands of Ukrainian peasants were therefore more than willing to uproot their families and accept an unbelievably generous Canadian government offer of a 160-acre homestead for only $10 (See Map 5 on page 14). Such an opportunity, glowingly described in government advertisements and praised in communications from fellow countrymen who had immigrated earlier, was too good to pass up. Many viewed this opportunity as God's reward for their suffering and undying faith. Others envisioned their new lives as soon equalling those of their wealthy landlords in the Old Country. Little could they know that this generous offer had as many hardships associated with it as the life they were leaving behind.

Entry into Canada required immigrants to be free of major health problems and to have adequate financial resources to be self-sufficient. Train travel from eastern Canadian ports quickly revealed the vastness and diversity of the Canadian landscape. The extensive forests and rocky terrain of Quebec and Ontario were distressing landscapes to the settlers, because such land was not suitable for agriculture. The more open southern regions of the western prairies, even though they had suitable farming soil, lacked significant forest cover and were also considered unattractive for settlement. A lack of trees meant an inadequate supply of building materials and firewood, which had been significant problems in the Old Country *(u kraiu)*.

The aspen parkland region (Map 3), a mixture of both wooded and grassland vegetation running through the central regions of the Prairie provinces, was seen as ideally suited to all their needs. This landscape closely resembled that of their homeland, and it contained numerous trees for building materials and fuel, grassy areas for animal forage, and rich black agricultural soil for growing crops. This wilderness, however, would require much sweat and tears before its bountiful potential could be realized. Fortunately, these early settlers possessed the prerequisites of success: patience, tolerance, perseverance, self-reliance, and the capacity for unlimited strenuous physical work.

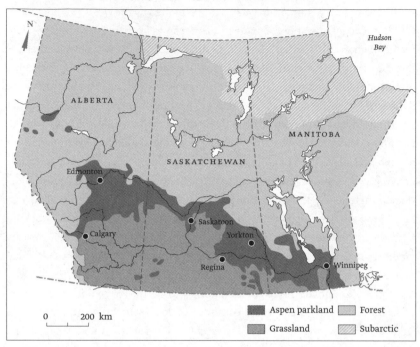

The federal government, to make the initial settlement process more successful, allowed the Ukrainian immigrants to create settlement blocs (Map 4). These were homestead areas with large concentrations of their countrymen, often related families or people from the same region or village in the Old Country. A common language and a strong sense of ethnic community helped ensure that neighbours not only helped one another, but readily shared their meagre resources. This socially isolating settlement pattern slowed the settlers' integration into Canadian society and generated considerable initial cultural and political resentment from Anglo-Saxon Canadians.

The first homestead dwellings were crude, sod-covered A-frame structures built over a pit. As soon as such a primitive dugout shelter *(burdei)* had been constructed, men often left their families on the undeveloped homestead and sought work elsewhere. Construction jobs in cities, as well as mine or railway work, became major sources of income to buy household supplies and

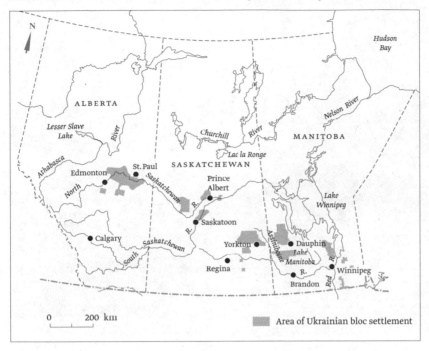

equipment. Women and children were left to begin clearing land for a small garden and a grain field. Isolation, in addition to the daily physical hardships, caused these women much sadness, anguish, suffering, and loneliness. In time functional farms developed, and growing families provided a workforce both on and off the farm. The income generated made it possible to purchase horses, ploughs, essential farm supplies, and even additional land.

As farm operations developed and prospered, other community-based needs and limitations became obvious. Lack of Ukrainian clergy and churches meant that religious rites (weddings, baptisms, funerals) were not being provided. Lack of rural schools severely limited educational opportunities for the children, even though education was viewed as the "door of opportunity" for the next generation. Concentration of doctors, dentists, druggists, and hospitals in distant cities and towns limited access to conventional health care practices. The additional burden of needing to pay for all medical

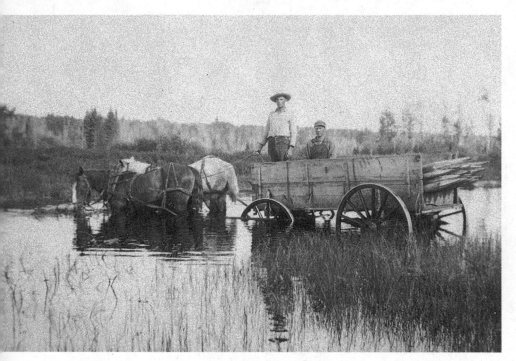

Ukrainian settlers sought out homesteads containing trees, grass, and water. [PAA UV652]

services and medications meant that these were not used much by cash-strapped settlers.

Bloc settlements supported the time-honoured and effective use of traditional Ukrainian home remedies and healing practices. These consisted of a variety of simple but effective treatments using household ingredients. Settlement areas were also home to traditional folk medicine practitioners, such as bonesetters and midwives, who provided more specialized services. In time, rural health care became more modernized as conventional medical services were made more accessible by better roads and means of transportation. Gradually, reliance on traditional health care practices and materials was replaced by more invasive and drug-based medical practices. Nevertheless, there is much to be learned and gained from knowing about the self-sufficiency of these folk healing traditions of the past. It is both the simplicity and effectiveness of these healing traditions and materials that I will describe in the pages that follow.

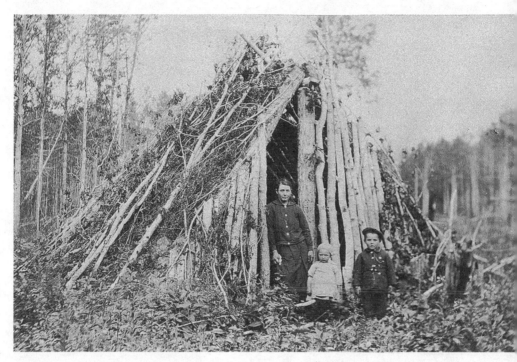

A log and mud hut *(burdei)*, the initial homestead shelter, was crude but functional. [PAA UV937]

# TWO

# Ancient Healing Practices

Historically, humans have discovered in nature, as have other animals, a variety of healing materials for treating illness, infection, and disease. These resources, widely available and easily used, are primarily plant materials, such as leaves, stems, roots, flowers, fruits, and seeds. As spiritual (religious) practices became a cultural element of human societies, illness and disease often became associated with evil spirits or vengeful deities. Certain members of society—the shamans, witch doctors, and medicine men and women—became recognized as traditional healers. Their healing practices, associated with supernatural elements, also relied heavily on the use of healing plant, animal, and mineral materials. Much of this traditional healing knowledge was derived from observing what plants sick animals ate, dream-based spiritual insights, and trial-and-error experimentation.

The Greeks were some of the first peoples to identify, evaluate, describe, and record the healing value of different plant species. Early on, they recognized 600 woody and non-woody plants as being medicinally helpful. The Greek physician Hippocrates expressed the importance of plants indirectly in his statement "Let food be your medicine and your medicine be your food."

Medicinal or herbal plants were often identifiable on the basis of such characteristics as a bitter flavour, strong odour, or irritating nature. They were also typically weedy species whose distribution corresponded to that of human activity, which became their major dispersal mechanism. The medicinal agents in these plants were naturally produced chemicals (secondary metabolites) that provided protection against herbivores and pests. These chemicals also proved to be extremely effective in treating a variety of human illnesses and diseases.

Aboriginal peoples also believe that the Creator has provided herbal treatments for every known human health problem, and that traditional healers could identify these relationships. Over time, healers developed individualized collections of secret preparations based on such natural materials, and they typically passed on their knowledge to worthy apprentices.

In time, with education becoming a significant social practice, traditional healing became less dependent on supernatural elements and more dependent on the knowledge of how to use a wide range of herbs. Egyptians in the West, and Indians and Chinese in the East, were some of the first peoples to effectively and widely study, describe, record, and use a wide variety of both cultivated and wild plants in their traditional folk medicine practices. The uses, preparations, and effectiveness of various folk treatments were preserved in their documents, but these records were limited in their availability and distribution. Oral transmission of folk medicine treatments remained the most effective way of spreading the knowledge, especially in the poorer and illiterate groups of society in which they were most used.

The Greeks and Romans were the first to formalize various healing traditions, and practitioners were required to serve apprenticeships before they were qualified to use them. These trained health practitioners eventually became known as physicians or doctors. The effectiveness of traditional medical treatments revealed that illnesses and diseases were organic (natural), rather than supernatural, in origin and could effectively be treated with natural materials, especially herbs. Human health was seen in a more holistic context and became associated with lifestyle features such as diet, hygiene, and living conditions. Fundamental Greek views on healing and health remained influential on Western medical developments and progress for more than a thousand years.

Western European trade and exploration led to the recognition that many other civilizations and Aboriginal peoples possessed distinctive and highly advanced traditional healing practices that also relied heavily on local, natural, and primarily herbal resources. This additional knowledge enriched, extended, and stimulated the formalization of the practice of herbalism throughout Europe. The Doctrine of Signatures, a spiritual concept of European origins but common to many Aboriginal peoples, became widely associated with herbal healing. The concept was based on the idea that God / the Creator provided humans with a diversity of healing plants, and their distinctive features were an indication of which body parts they influenced. Walnuts were to be used for brain disorders, beans for kidney ailments, etc. The development of the printing press in the fifteenth century resulted in production and widespread distribution of herbal publications (Herbals), which made such knowledge more available and more widely applied. The scientific study of plants, known as botany, has historically been associated with the rise and advancement of scientific medicine. By the sixteenth century, often referred to as the Age of Herbalism, the number of recognized medicinally useful plants was in the thousands, and herbal publications were widely popular. Monasteries became not only the centres of herbal knowledge, but also maintained healing gardens and provided health care to the poor and needy.

By the seventeenth century, Western-based health practices were becoming more scientific and associated with formalized education, which distanced them from traditional folk medicine practices. Conventional medical practices became more dependent on chemically based medicines and used a variety of invasive surgical treatments. Medical practice required university-based education and training; was dominated by male practitioners; and became highly commercialized in the urban setting, where it was concentrated. Traditional or folk medicine continued to serve the poor and uneducated rural masses and became primarily associated with uneducated female practitioners, often labelled witches or medicine women. Common folk, those of the poorly educated lower classes in society, typically distrusted the new scientific medical practice and could not afford its services. Growing popularity of folk medicine among the masses soon came to be seen by physicians as a threat to their prosperity and prestige. Various forms of legislation were introduced to severely limit traditional medicine's availability and practice, but it nevertheless survived in the form of "household" or "kitchen" medicine and was passed on from mother to daughter as a way of meeting family health needs.

The popularity of traditional healing practices was associated with their widespread availability, simplicity, relatively safety, cost effectiveness, and use in dealing with wide variety of simple and common ailments. To this day it has retained many of its original features and has developed into a variety of alternative medical therapies, which are seen by many as a highly desirable complement to conventional medicine.

It was this traditional folk medicine, widely practised in rural areas of the Old Country that became a major source of comfort and relief to the early Ukrainian settlers as they found themselves struggling to survive in the isolated backwoods of western Canada. Using Baba's kitchen medicine, passed on from generation to generation, they could effectively deal with most of the family's daily health needs. This knowledge also became a part of the community "fabric," strengthening cultural connections by making people more dependent on one another.

# Ukrainian Folk Healing Traditions

Early Ukrainian settlers were familiar with both conventional (practised in urban settings) and traditional (practised in rural settings) healing practices. In the Old Country, most of the latest medical advances, knowledge, and resources were available in cities and towns, but small and isolated rural villages relied for the most part on traditional folk medicine, which was distinctly regional and localized. Ukrainians living in Bukovina, a less-developed region of Ukraine, practised a more diverse and native-plant-based folk medicine tradition. People living in Galicia, a more developed region, relied more on the use of cultivated plant materials and local household products in their home remedies. Villages, and even families, had their own distinctive variations on healing treatments and materials. What initially might appear to be a wide diversity of treatments for similar conditions is often nothing more than a narrow range of treatments with a degree of variation. Village priests were generally some of the better educated individuals and were often sought out for advice in treating the more serious health conditions. They were also legally permitted to possess alcohol, which was a widely used ingredient for tincture-based home remedies. Priests recognized when it was necessary to send a patient to the city for a doctor's treatment and therefore provided villagers with a broader range of medical possibilities.

In Ukrainian settlement blocs throughout western Canada, isolation and harsh environmental conditions became significant challenges to staying healthy. Clearing and maintaining a homestead required extremely hard and even dangerous physical labour. Many daily household and farming activities

MAP 5   Allocation of free homestead lands in a township

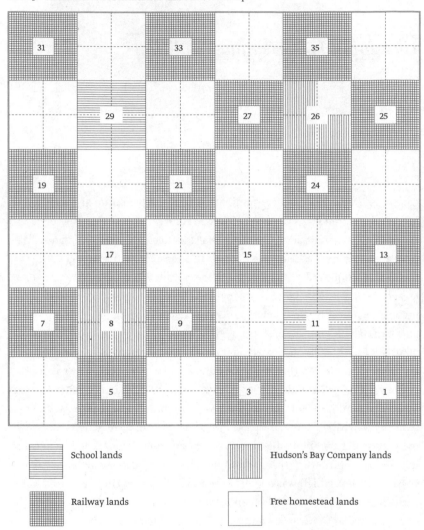

| | | | | | |
|---|---|---|---|---|---|
| School lands | | | Hudson's Bay Company lands | | |
| Railway lands | | | Free homestead lands | | |

*Plan of a typical township showing: (a) school lands (sections 11 and 29, (b) Hudson's Bay Company lands (section 8 and three-quarters of section 26; the whole of 26 in every fifth township, (c) free homestead lands (even-numbered sections, except 8 and 26), (d) railway lands (odd-numbered sections reserved for selection as railway land grants). Each section is bounded on three sides by road allowances (66 feet).*

were equally strenuous and hazardous, resulting in accidents and sometimes serious injuries. Overcrowded and stuffy living conditions in relatively primitive dwellings, poor hygiene, a lack of adequate sanitation, and seasonal dietary limitations meant that illness was an ever-present threat to everyone, but especially a concern of the very young and very old. Initially, a lack of rural doctors and hospitals was the major impediment to accessing outside health care, but cost factors and a deep suspicion of conventional medicine's invasive practices continued to limit its use by the Ukrainians for anything but the most serious medical problems.

*One of my fingers* (paltsi) *developed an abnormal reddish growth, and I suffered with it for three weeks before I went to the doctor. He wanted to amputate the finger, but I begged him not to. He cut off the growth but it returned in a week or so. I wrapped coltsfoot* (pidbil) *on the affected finger and it not only reduced the pain but also drew out whatever was in the growth. When I went back to the doctor, he noticed the plant material under the bandage and said, "Ukrainians are crazy* (variiaty)." *He cleaned out the finger again; it healed, and I still have my finger to this day.* — M. M. / Edmonton

Ukrainian homesteaders were generally medically self-reliant and used a range of traditional home healing practices and materials. Women, being generally more sensitive and caring in nature, were typically the family's health care providers. They readily shared their knowledge of traditional healing treatments and materials with family, friends, and neighbours. This "socialized" the community's medical care and made people more interdependent. Traditional healing practices, never rigidly formalized, were also continuously changing and adapting to the availability of local healing resources. If a widely used treatment proved less effective, it was readily modified with other ingredients, incorporated store-bought and patented products, or integrated with other healing approaches.

*Home remedies were shared, by word of mouth, from one person to another.*
*People from different Ukrainian settlement areas exchanged treatments and*
*remedies that had been used in their home villages. Women were the most*
*interested in these practices, and the older women* (starshi zhinky) *were the*
*ones who knew the most. They were the ones in the area who were really helpful in*
*treating and healing the sick and were called upon as necessary.* — M. M. / Lamont

The family's health and well-being, generally under the mother's care, was supplemented with the advice and experience of the community's grandmothers. Such elderly wisdom was much sought out, especially if the condition was serious or if the healer was young and inexperienced. Such home-based treatments were in most cases sufficient to deal with daily cuts, bruises, seasonal colds, and related minor conditions. In situations where the home remedy or treatment proved ineffective, especially when the patient was a child, a mother's loving care and concern helped alleviate the sense of hopelessness in the situation. Often just keeping the child calm and comforted was sufficient to allow natural healing processes to take their course. Strong faith, associated with prayer and a belief in divine intervention, also provided both patient and caregiver with additional comfort, strength, and support in trying times.

Available Ukrainian- or English-language newspapers, magazines, and publications that targeted rural communities were additional sources of health-related information. Papers and magazines often contained shared personal testimonials, by people of various ethnic backgrounds, of effective home remedies and treatments.

Nuns of various religious orders were often located in larger Ukrainian settlement areas. They functioned much like the village priests in the Old Country by providing both conventional and traditional health care advice. Later on, as public schools became more widespread, the teacher similarly became an invaluable source of knowledge on modern hygiene practices and health-related information. Language barriers, as well as the practice of establishing bloc settlements, limited the exchange of healing treatments and materials between Ukrainians, other ethnic groups, and Aboriginal peoples. In many cases where settlements were located near reserves, Aboriginal people were sought out for their medicines, and these were openly shared.

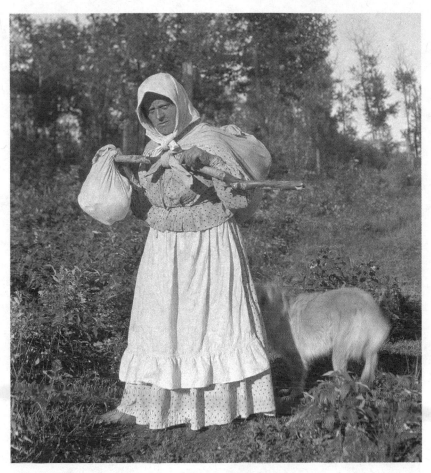

Mother was the family healer and a community resource. [PAM N11601]

*A man suffered from asthma* (iadukha), *and the doctors were not able to help him. While he was at a powwow on a reserve in the area, he started coughing heavily. An Indian man looked at him and said that it sounded serious and could kill him if it was not treated. He told him to go into the forest* (lis) *when he got home and to cut off a few spruce* (ialyna) *branches. One large branch was to be placed in each corner of the house and the branches were to be replaced when they dried out and were no longer fragrant. He did this for a month and was totally cured of his condition. To this day he has no troubles with his breathing.* — M. K. / Smoky Lake

Traditional Ukrainian folk medicine associates illness with physical (body) or emotional (mind) disruption of the body's inner balance or harmony. This imbalance may occur as a result of biological agents (parasites), physical factors (heat), dietary features (lack of fibre), or work-related issues (heavy lifting). In many cases, the condition of the person's blood was considered to be a major contributing factor to poor health. "Bad" blood *(paskudna krov)* was often removed by means of bloodletting, cupping (wet), or application of leeches. Traditional cures for physical ailments varied greatly, and treatments ranged widely among folk healers. Conditions with an emotional basis (fear, sleeplessness) were considered to be of a spiritual nature and were treated almost exclusively by spiritual healers. These individuals, mainly elderly women, used wax pouring *(visk zlyvaty)* or similar divination techniques to assist the patient in overcoming their difficulties. Their success was well known, and their services were in demand throughout the community.

The wide range of traditional healing resources served the community's health needs effectively in the early days of settlement and also continued to be used well after doctors and hospitals became more widely available. These folk healing practices began to decline only after the younger generations became more educated and absorbed into Canadian culture and practices. Young people were unwilling, for fear of being ridiculed, to continue being treated with crude home-based remedies because these were considered primitive and "ethnic." Embarrassment, and not ineffectiveness, contributed to the widespread decrease in their use. Nevertheless, even to this day, many of these old-time home remedies are fondly remembered, and some continue to be used by elderly Ukrainians who nostalgically recall them from their childhood. I am confident in saying that most readers of this book have either experienced some type of traditional healing practice themselves, know of someone who has used them, or at least heard them spoken about at family gatherings. We may yet see the time when household "kitchen medicine" is revived as a desirable and widespread practice to be used with self-sufficient pride and not naïve embarrassment.

# FOUR

# Healers in Ukrainian Settlements

Ukrainian settlements typically had a variety of specialized traditional healers. The most important ones were the bonesetter, who treated dislocations and broken bones in both humans and animals and could also pull teeth; the midwife *(povytukha)*, who assisted with pregnancy and childbirth; and the spiritual healer, who poured wax to treat emotional problems. Often such a healer was identified as a medicine man or woman, a faith healer, a witch, an old woman *(baba)*, an old man *(dido)*, a plant "doctor" (herbalist), or an animal "doctor." Some healers made use of both natural (herbs) and supernatural (prayers, invocations) elements in their treatments. The latter made their services more tolerated and accepted by the church. I was told of numerous examples where medical doctors, unable to treat a health problem successfully, referred their patient to an appropriate traditional healer who successfully treated the person. Often, people went to their traditional healers when doctors recommended amputation as the medical course of action.

Within the family, the grandmother was most often involved in the use and application of home remedies and treatments. Women born in Canada learned their use by watching others, or would have had this matriarchal knowledge passed on by a mother or other female relative.

> My elderly aunt (titka) *was the local healer in our area, and many people went to her for help. Even the town doctor sent her patients. She knew how to apply cups* (banky) *and leeches* (p'iavky) *to remove "bad" blood* (paskudna krov). *This blood usually collected in the lower part of the back or kidney region and caused*

*a bad aching pain. My aunt would make fine cuts on the skin, in the area that
ached, and then place the cups over these in order to remove the "bad" blood. This
blood was very dark in colour. It could also be removed with the use of leeches.*
— S. S. / Camrose


Monetary payment for such services was traditionally not expected and in
most cases was not possible. Patient gratitude was most often expressed with
"local currency," which consisted of produce, eggs, meat, moonshine, or some
other farm product. Spiritual healers especially, because of the religious nature
of the treatment, were never paid directly since their ability to heal was believed
to be a divine gift to be used for the betterment of society. Nevertheless, a payment was often expected and was left behind without being given directly to
the healer.

A widespread practice in many Ukrainian homes was the illegal production of whisky *(horivka)* or homebrew *(samohonka).* These highly potent alcoholic
preparations were used in a large variety of traditional remedies and treatments.
Prohibition in the early 1900s made it difficult for people to obtain alcohol—
it was legally available only from druggists when prescribed by a doctor. It is
not surprising that many such prescriptions were written and that some of
this alcohol was used for other than medicinal purposes. Homebrew was preferred for medicinal use because it was more potent, especially if it was distilled
twice. The second distillation was often identified as "medicinal whisky," and
a jar of it was typically kept in a home just for such use. It was also common
knowledge who, in a settlement area, could provide such an effective and
widely used home remedy if a person's own supply ran out. Its use was mainly
reserved for adults. If administered to children, it was dispensed in teaspoon or
tablespoon portions.


## BONESETTERS

The majority of bonesetters were male, which suggests that such skills may have
been developed with paramedical training received during a man's compulsory
three-year service in the Austro-Hungarian military. Female practitioners would

most likely have been taught this skill by a father or male relative. In some cases, an untrained bonesetter believed that the talent was a "divine" gift and simply refined it with experience.

> *The bonesetter in our area was so good that even the local doctor* (likar) *sent him patients with broken bones and sprained joints. He had no training in it, but said it was a gift from God* (Boh) *that he had. He would feel the injured area, and if it was only a dislocation he would twist it back. If it was a break, he would set the bones* (kosti skladaty), *put on a splint, and then bandage it.* — P. N. / Lamont

Bonesetters mainly treated sprains, dislocations, crushed digits, and broken bones. Some even extended such treatment to similar conditions in large animals. A few bonesetters were also proficient in dealing with "bad" teeth and extracted them with pliers. If a settlement area did not have a bonesetter, an injured person might resort to self-treatment for a simple injury such as a sprain, fracture, or simple break. More serious bone injuries required the services of a doctor and a possible stay in the hospital, both of which were costly.

Injuries, if simple and the patient was mobile, were treated at the bonesetter's home, but if the person was immobilized and the injury serious, the bonesetter came to the patient's home. The swollen limb might initially be soaked in hot whey (liquid residue from cheese production) or an Epsom salts solution to reduce the swelling. It was then set, by means of gentle but effective manipulation, and stabilized by means of thin wooden boards *(doshky)*. The splints may have been brought over from the Old Country, but could also be made out of white poplar *(topolia)* wood or even bark. These were bound in place with strips of linen cloth or pieces of hemp rope, which, if covered with egg white, formed a crude cast. A sling might also be improvised, from a kerchief or piece of cloth, to reduce strain on the injured area. Most often the injury healed well; the service matched any results a medical doctor might provide and certainly was less costly. Injuries treated by a less-skilled bonesetter, or by the injured person themself, could be less successful. Permanent disfiguration of the limb often led to life-long crippling.

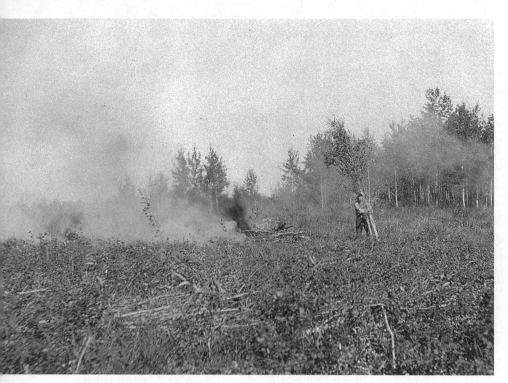

Clearing the homestead, which was hard and hazardous work, required everyone's contribution. [PAA UV938]

*In our area, my uncle* (vuiko) *was the bonesetter, but he had no formal training in it. His daughter broke her collarbone in school* (shkola) *and he set and bandaged it completely. He took her to a doctor a few weeks later to see how it was healing. The doctor said it was perfect job, but then got mad because a common man could do such good work and was probably causing him to lose money. The doctor was partly right, because people came from miles around for my uncle's services but he never charged people for his work.* — C. S. / Edmonton

## MIDWIVES

In the early settlement period, families were often quite large—having ten or more children was common. Assistance at a baby's birth was most often provided by the local midwife. She was generally an elderly woman who had either been taught these skills by another midwife, was self-taught and experienced, or simply was someone who had given birth to a number of children and knew what to expect. Midwives were highly valued because of their skills and experience, and vital to a community's well-being and growth. Successful deliveries, in some cases numbering over a hundred, greatly refined their skills and knowledge. Such experienced help was much appreciated by a doctor during a difficult home delivery. Doctors and hospitals, primarily because of their cost, were used only if the pregnancy was difficult, if there was a prolonged period of labour, or if the delivery was expected to be risky.

A midwife typically served a specific area and tried not to overlap with others in the district. Familiarity and trust were important elements to an expectant mother, especially if it was her first delivery. A midwife's services were provided at any time and under all types of conditions. Her involvement both reassured and comforted the expectant mother, especially if her husband was working away from home and if family, relatives, or friends were unavailable. In situations where an experienced midwife was not available, a female relative, a neighbour, or even the husband could be called on to provide birthing assistance.

A midwife, notified of the expected delivery date, would come a few days earlier to help organize the household and make preparations for the birth. She might even take on some basic household responsibilities for a few days before—and in some cases a few days after—the delivery, to give the mother much-needed rest. She often brought her own supply of traditional preparations for both the mother and baby. These might include compounds to numb and sterilize any necessary birthing cuts or tears, alcohol as an antiseptic, infusions to strengthen and relax the woman, goose fat to keep tissues supple and initiate healing, and an infusion to clear up and strengthen the newborn's digestive system. If the mother's membranes did not break naturally, the midwife might need to induce delivery by breaking them. She would tie off the umbilical cord with any available material, sometimes resorting to binder twine if nothing else was at hand. The baby would be cleaned up and washed before being passed to the mother. If the placenta was not expelled naturally, the midwife might attempt to remove it manually. Only when she knew that the mother and baby could be safely left on their own, and that household chores were being looked after, did she return home to her own accumulated work. Many of my informants were living testimonials to the effectiveness and success of such capable women.

## SPIRITUAL HEALERS

These specialized healers, typically elderly women, used divine (Jesus, Virgin Mary) intervention in their healing practices. Because of their reclusive, eccentric, or secretive nature, as well as the fact that their ability was considered a spiritual "gift," they were often referred to as witches *(vorozhka / chaklunka / vidma)*. They nevertheless were much respected in their community and were certainly widely used. Over 80 per cent of my informants said that they knew of their services, either directly (having received treatment themselves) or indirectly (knowing someone who had been treated). Treatment was sought if the affected person showed prolonged signs of anxiety, fear *(strakh)*, sleeplessness, general nervousness, or tension. A few of these women also provided non-spiritual treatments for physical ailments, which used various plant and animal ingredients.

The most common healing practice was based on special prayers, incantations, and blessings. These were used in conjunction with some blessed object, such as water, wax, or a knife, which provided a visible physical element to the healing ritual. The treatment, applied over three separate occasions, was generally successful and further enhanced the healer's reputation. Because of the religious nature of this treatment, it was widely tolerated by the local churches. A Sister of a Ukrainian religious order in Edmonton said it channelled the healing powers of God and therefore did not go against church beliefs or practices. This healing tradition continues to be used in Ukrainian communities today and has been well documented in Alberta by Rina Hanchuk's 1999 publication *The Word and Wax* (see Selected Readings).

> *An older person in our area poured wax to heal sick* (slabi) *people. She had the person sit in a chair, held a bowl of holy/blessed water* (sviachena voda) *over their head, and then while praying poured melted wax into the water. The*

*image formed by the wax allowed her to "see" what was the cause of the person's*
*condition. She then continued praying* (molytysia) *for the person to be healed.*
— E. L. / Two Hills


## HERBALISTS

These individuals, sometimes referred to as "plant doctors," would have had
formal training in the use of different healing plants *(likarski roslyny)*. They were
typically men, and were common practitioners in the Old Country. Some may
well have been trained as naturopathic doctors, which gave them the designation "doctor." They were, however, extremely rare in Ukrainian bloc settlements,
and very few of my informants were aware of such individuals in their home
community. These men would have had little incentive to emigrate, since they
would not have been farmers and would typically have practised in urban areas.
Those who immigrated to Canada would probably have set up practices, along
with the naturopaths, in larger towns and cities.

Rural areas with a strong Eastern European population base were, however,
served on an irregular basis by such urban-based herbalists and naturopaths.
These healers, like the Watkins or Rawleigh salesmen who sold both patent
medicines and various herbs, made visits to these settlement areas throughout
the year. They provided highly specialized services and products such as herbal
preparations, cupping, and leeches. Herbs and herbal preparations were also
available by mail order through advertisements in magazines and newspapers,
or from catalogues (Eaton's).


*There was an herbal healer in our area, and he had been trained as a naturopath*
*in the Old Country. Mother used to take us to him when she did not know what*
*to do for our problem. He treated my brother's eczema* (vysypka) *with a dark*
*ointment* (maz), *and it healed well. Since he was not licensed to work in the*
*province, he did not advertise and only helped people who came to him. He would*
*not accept money* (hroshi) *for his help but was "paid" with farm products.*
*My mother learned a lot from him, because she was very interested in natural*
*remedies and healing.* — C. O. / Edmonton

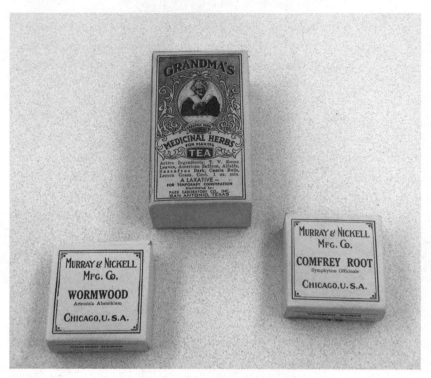

Packaged medicinal herbs were available from a variety of sources. [M. MUCZ]

Rural areas did have individuals who had no formal training in the use of healing plants, but had the knowledge passed on to them by a family member or by someone who developed their own interests in this practice. Such persons, again mainly men, were also not common. They may have brought seeds and cuttings of healing plants with them from the Old Country, grown them in Canada, and provided their resources and knowledge to those who came to them for help. They would also have discovered that many of the healing plants that they were familiar with, commonly weeds, were also found in Canada. Most of the plants used in traditional Ukrainian healing practices were domesticated species and were grown in gardens and fields on any homestead. Unfortunately, language barriers, as well as general lack of interaction with Aboriginal people *(andiiany)*, prevented the settlers from learning about the healing potential of many native plants.

## DOCTORS AND DENTISTS

In the early settlement period, professional health care services from doctors, dentists, and druggists were seldom available in rural areas. "There were no doctors *(ne bulo doktoriv)*" was a comment I often heard from my informants. This undoubtedly resulted in many unnecessary deaths on isolated home-steads and forced families to rely on traditional home-based folk remedies and treatments.

> *Many people would have died* (povmyraly) *if there were no such things as home remedies. Mothers were the home doctors and saved* (vriatuvaly) *many people.*
> — A. W. / Daysland

As professional (paid) medical care became more available, health care cost became a significant concern because all medical expenses were the direct responsibility of the patient. In the early 1900s, an eleven-day stay in a hospital to deliver a baby, including a doctor's services, cost $38. A regular house call to a homestead cost $2 to $5, and for maternity cases, the charge increased to $15 to $23. A travelling charge of $1 per mile was also added to the bill. An appendix operation, requiring a seven-day hospital stay, would seriously strain cash-poor household budgets. Medical payments to town doctors were often made with the "local currency": meat, dairy products, produce, baking, firewood, or labour. This kept the doctor comfortable and well fed, but cash poor.

The farther a homestead was from town, the less likely it was that its family could access, let alone afford, medical services. Isolation and cost forced many families to rely on patent medicines such as Aspirin, cod liver oil, ointments, and liniments, which they purchased from travelling salesmen or mail-order catalogues (Eaton's in Winnipeg). Do-it-yourself medical manuals, such as various "doctor" books, also described a range of treatments for common, non-life-threatening health problems. Even when a doctor's services were more access-ible, they were typically called upon only after various home treatments had failed. Often this meant that the medical condition was more aggravated than if the patient had sought treatment earlier. Doctors often became frustrated with their patients when they found out about the folk treatments they had been using, which they considered to be crude, primitive practices.

> *A woman had stepped on a hay fork, and soon her foot* (stopa) *became so infected that she could not walk. Even though the doctor was treating the infection* (zaraza), *the leg was not healing and was becoming more swollen. A neighbour came by and said she knew what could be done to have her walking the next day. She went into the pasture and collected some fresh cow manure* (hnii vid korovy). *She put it on a cloth and wrapped it around the infected foot. In the morning, when the doctor came by, he was amazed as to how well the leg was healing. When he asked the woman what she had done to get it healing so well, she was too embarrassed to tell him and said nothing.* — A. C. / Mundare

The medical knowledge and drugs of the day were also limited and in many cases not very effective. Many health conditions, such as diabetes, were poorly understood and treatments were inadequate and uncertain. It was with some justification that many of the older settlers were suspicious of conventional medical knowledge and in many cases disturbed by its reliance on invasive (surgical) and drug-based (chemical) treatments. Amputation was a commonly suggested treatment for injured limbs, fingers, or toes. A doctor's services were used, however, for treating more serious conditions such as an inflamed appendix or tonsils, a difficult pregnancy or delivery, or a serious injury.

Early on, language was a major barrier to communicating about health problems with a doctor. Doctors who understood or spoke Ukrainian, often Jewish, were more trusted and sought out, especially by the elderly. Often it was extremely difficult for the patient to come to the doctor, and a seventy-kilometre ride into town by horse-drawn wagon might require a full day's journey. Making a house call was critical for seriously ill patients, and neither time, distance, nor bad weather were insurmountable obstacles to rural practitioners. These trips were made on horseback or by buggy in summer and by horse-drawn cutter in winter. In his town office, often a part of his home, the doctor's wife was not only his nursing assistant but also the receptionist and hostess for his out-of-town

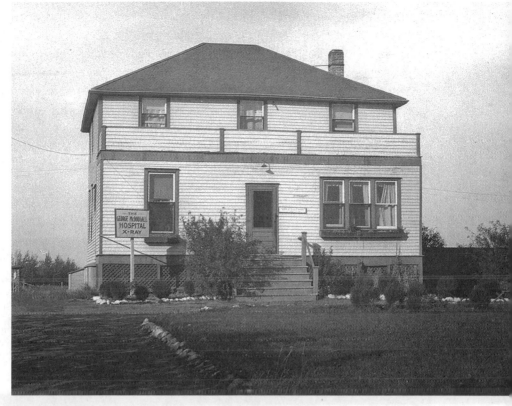

Hospitals, if available in the area, were expensive and only used as a last resort. [PAA G363]

patients. For many such couples medicine was truly a family affair, and patient care often extended beyond the office and into the household.

Rotating "clinics" also visited rural schools to evaluate the general health of students and provide surgery for inflamed tonsils. An area of the school was curtained off for surgery, and another area had cots for pupils coming out of the anesthetic.

> *Kids packed all kinds of things into their ears (vukho). During a school health checkup the doctor would pull out pussy willows, pencil lead, and other things from students' ears.* — T. B. / Edmonton

Dentists were uncommon in small towns at the beginning of the twentieth century, and doctors typically received dental training (anesthesia, extraction, etc.) in their final year of medical school. In small-town practices, doctors also provided basic dental services, such as extractions. The charge for pulling a tooth was $1. In more isolated regions, a doctor and a dentist would regularly visit towns that had no permanent medical services and provided essential surgical (tonsil removal) and dental procedures.

Most rural communities did not have a drugstore, and doctors often served as druggist by dispensing the prescribed medications. Such additional dental and pharmaceutical practices provided much-needed supplementary income for doctors. These services also meant better overall health care for patients, which in time contributed to the decline in use of home remedies and treatments. The Canadian-born generation of Ukrainians slowly lost faith in traditional healing and enthusiastically embraced scientific medicine.

# FIVE

# Homestead Health Concerns

## GENERAL PROBLEMS

Homestead life was hard to begin with and was further stressed by accidents, illnesses, and contagious diseases. During the early period of settlement, families often had to live in crude, stuffy, and cramped living quarters; possessed inadequate winter clothing and footwear; practised limited personal hygiene; had the crudest sanitation facilities; used the most basic food preparation and preservation techniques; and had an extremely restricted diet, especially over the winter. These conditions, in various combinations, led to health problems, especially in the very young, the very old, and those weakened by chronic illness. Most often the sick person could do no more than suffer *(terpity)* through their condition, but this was difficult for children, who wanted immediate comfort and relief. For adults, common injuries and infections were caused by axe, scythe, sickle, and even gunshot wounds. Breaks, fractures, and bone-crushing injuries occurred while clearing land, working with large animals or farm equipment, or doing other hazardous farm work. Strained muscles and sore backs were a regular result of physically strenuous work. All such injuries were treated, with differing degrees of effectiveness, using kitchen medicine. Such traditional home healing was well suited for common, everyday health problems, but of less value in dealing with more serious conditions such as broken bones, breathing difficulties, or chronic illnesses. Only when healing with home remedies was ineffective, or when the condition worsened, did families resort to seeking professional medical help.

*God walked with us that day as my daughter (dochka) and I made our way along a freshly cut path. My child (dytyna) suddenly cried out in pain and I could see that she had stepped on a sharp piece of branch. The wood had gone right through her foot, and I could see the blood-covered wood sticking out near her toes. I had nothing with which I could pull out the branch, so I lay her down and carefully lifted her foot to my mouth. I grasped the branch with my teeth (zuby) and gently pulled it out and then wrapped the wound. I carried my daughter home and then soaked her foot in warm water. The wound was kept wrapped in cloth and it healed well.*
— S. R. / Smoky Lake

## CHILDREN'S PROBLEMS

Children's natural curiosity, inexperience, carelessness, and boldness meant that they were more likely to suffer accidental injuries. Burns, cuts, scrapes, and puncture wounds were almost daily occurrences in young children playing in and exploring the farm setting. Broken or sprained limbs, from falls, heavy labour, or working around farm animals and machinery, were not uncommon in the older children.

*When I was five years old, I was playing with an older girl (divchynka) who was spinning me around by my hands. When she let me go, I fell down and dislocated my hand. Mother took me to an old man who knew how to set bones. He made me soak my hand in warm whey for an hour (na hodynu). He then adjusted it and wrapped it up. My hand healed well, and I have not had any problems with it to this day (do sohodni).* — M. S. / Vegreville

Childhood illnesses such as measles, mumps, and chicken pox were unpredictable but expected and were also treated with folk medicine. Other illnesses such as diphtheria, typhoid, scarlet fever, whooping cough, consumption (tuberculosis), cholera, and smallpox required medical intervention, which could result in a costly hospital stay. Untreated pneumonia and appendicitis were life-threatening conditions that also required immediate medical attention —which was often unavailable or difficult to access.

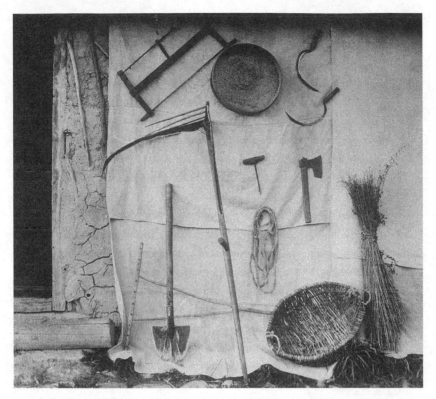

Sharp tools were used daily and contributed to many serious injuries [film image]

School teachers *(uchytel)* played a major role in children's well-being and often had to deal directly (treatment) or indirectly (send home) with infectious problems such as head lice or skin conditions (ringworm, itch). Children who had been exposed to the more serious and contagious diseases, such as chicken pox, measles, and scarlet fever, were sent home, and the teacher was required to inform the municipal health authority of the situation. This could result in the family's homestead being quarantined, which meant that visiting and leaving the house were not permitted until the illness was no longer considered contagious. Sometimes such a quarantine order could last a month or more, causing real hardship for the family. Under such circumstances, people attempted to make the household environment less contagious by fumigating it by burning sulphur in a pail.

*Children* (dity) *who had head lice* (vushi) *would pass them to others in school.*
*When the Sisters [nuns] came to teach at our school, they called a meeting to*
*deal with the problem. Parents had to buy a special comb* (hrebin) *with fine teeth*
*on both sides. My mother combed my hair with it all the time. If the Sisters found*
*a student with lice, they cut their hair short and then rubbed kerosene on it. A*
*paper bag was put over the hair and the student had to sit in class with it on.*
*This was done for a few days and it helped clear up the school lice problem.*
— J. L. / Mundare


## EMOTIONAL PROBLEMS

Endless physical work, large families, inadequate financial and material resources, homesickness, and isolation caused significant daily stress in people's lives.
Additionally, long distances between neighbours, demands of daily life, and language barriers greatly reduced opportunities for social interaction. This deprived
depressed individuals of support, understanding, and relief from their over-
whelming feelings of despair. Such accumulated pressures, over time, often created emotional problems in vulnerable individuals, especially in women. Bouts
of depression, hysteria, nervousness, shaking, nausea, hallucinations, fatigue,
lethargy, sleeplessness, or feelings of poor self-worth were common symptoms
of their distress. Medical care for such emotional problems was not readily available or advanced enough to be very effective, and most such problems became a
guarded family secret.

Women were probably the most emotionally affected by such isolation and
lack of socialization. They rarely left the homestead, whereas men could social-
ize in town when doing various chores and the children interacted with others
at school. The monotonous routines of daily farm and household tasks took
their toll on the emotional well-being of women. Frequent pregnancies, raising
infants, and caring for numerous children were physically and emotionally challenging. Opportunities for comfort and relief from such stresses were limited to
small periods of quiet time in the evening when things became more settled.
This meant that visits and religious events were eagerly anticipated and much
enjoyed occasions. Alcohol abuse, especially by men who made homebrew, was
a common problem and often led to emotional and physical abuse in the family.

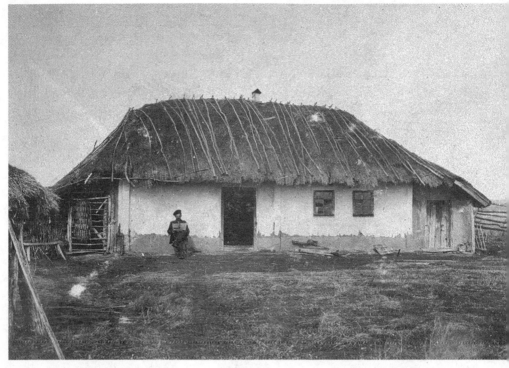
Old Country styles, customs, and traditions characterized Ukrainian prairie homesteads. [PAA UV4]

Children, in particular, were easily traumatized by fearful and unexpected experiences. Encounters with wild animals, being chased by aggressive farm animals, meeting strangers, or having a bad accident were potentially traumatic events for them. Such experiences could easily lead to prolonged periods of nervousness, fussiness, crying, general agitation, poor eating, fitful sleep, and bedwetting.

A typical folk medicine diagnosis was to associate these symptoms with some supernatural and consuming fear. Being bewitched (*navrochuvaty*) by the evil eye (*uroky*), cast through the look of an envious individual, could make a person lethargic, anxious, and experience excessive sweating. Even animals could become bewitched, and this resulted in their having a run-down appearance, showing a change in feeding habits, or declining in health until they died.

The prevailing cultural view was that such conditions had supernatural origins, and medical help would be of little use. Conventional medicine at the time was limited in the treatments it could provide to improve mental health. Doctors tended to send such patients to traditional healers for help, often with positive results. Treatment, based on "pouring off the fright" *(zlyvaty strakh),* was available from a spiritual folk healer—an older person or someone identified as a "witch" who possessed the appropriate healing ability. These individuals knew how to pour wax or throw coals *(vuhlia skydaty)* to effect a cure and were often successful (see section on spiritual healing in chapter eight).

*I came home from a dance and was sweating and not feeling well. My mother said that someone had cast the "evil eye" on me because I was a good-looking young man* (molodyi cholovik). *She said she knew what to do to cure it. A little later on she came up behind me, suddenly grabbed and turned me around, and sprayed a mouthful of water [holy water?] all over my face. I slept well that night and felt much better the next day.* — M. L. / Edmonton

# SIX

# Health Conditions Treated

Traditional folk medicine sees illness as a loss of inner balance, or harmony, in the body (physical) or the mind (emotional). This might result from biological (parasites), physical (injury), dietary, or lifestyle changes. In the early days, microbial pathogens (flu virus) and physiological ailments (diabetes) were poorly understood, even by conventional medicine, and their treatments were rudimentary at best. Each physical illness is typically identified with a distinctive set of symptoms (cough, fever) that determine the nature of the treatment required. Since many symptoms are not exclusive to one disorder and overlap considerably, home-based treatments attempted to address the symptoms to cure the condition. This is why many different conditions were treated with similar household ingredients used in similar applications.

Natural remedies for simple health problems were, in most cases, quite effective, or at least made the sick person feel better and allowed the body's natural healing processes to take their course. More complex and involved physical treatments using manipulation or specialized applications (cups) required the services of specialized folk healers, such as bonesetters and midwives (see descriptions in chapter four). Treatment of emotional problems required an element of spiritual intervention provided by a spiritual healer (described in chapter eight).

The elderly considered the condition of the blood, which maintained all the body tissues and organs, as a major indicator of physical well-being. The concept of "bad" blood was therefore associated with poor health. This meant that it had to be removed by means of bloodletting, cupping (wet), or the use of leeches, which were all features of folk healing practices.

TABLE 2    Medical conditions and types treated with home remedies

| Medical Condition | Condition Types Treated | Informant Responses |
|---|---|---|
| Skin | 15 | 1,268 |
| Head (ear, eye, nose) | 7 | 836 |
| Gastrointestinal and liver | 10 | 598 |
| Respiratory | 5 | 371 |
| General health | 7 | 310 |
| Musculoskeletal | 6 | 308 |
| Circulatory and urinary | 4 | 192 |
| Common diseases | 6 | 62 |
| Female conditions | 3 | 39 |
| **Total** | **63** | **3,984** |

TABLE 3    Variety of home treatments and materials used for skin conditions

| Medical Condition | Treatments and Materials Used | Informant Use |
|---|---|---|
| Wounds (infected) | 41 | 221 |
| Burns | 36 | 113 |
| Boils | 35 | 165 |
| Rashes | 31 | 100 |
| Ringworm | 28 | 43 |
| Cuts (bleeding) | 24 | 139 |
| Chapped skin | 21 | 146 |
| Puncture wounds | 20 | 110 |
| Warts | 20 | 42 |
| Wounds (healing) | 20 | 67 |
| Frozen skin | 17 | 55 |
| Diaper rash | 15 | 49 |
| Insect bites | 7 | 14 |
| Slivers | 2 | 2 |
| Fleas and mites | 2 | 2 |
| **Total** | **319** | **1,268** |

This study found informants describing almost 4,000 individual healing situations that used traditional healing remedies or practices (Table 2). It also identified sixty-three specific health conditions or illnesses that were treated with such kitchen medicine. Almost two thirds of the described treatments were associated with skin, head, or gastrointestinal problems, and over 50 per cent of the different health problems treated were related to these body parts. Common diseases and female health developments were the least described and treated of all conditions. Most diseases were too serious to be treated by folk remedies and required a doctor's attention. Female concerns were seldom openly discussed, because cultural and gender barriers made it difficult for informants to address such topics comfortably with a man, let alone with a stranger.

The number of different separate home-based treatments described for various medical conditions varied from as few as twenty-six for common diseases (Table 10), which were typically treated by a doctor, to as many as 319 for skin problems (Table 3). The skin, the body's largest organ, is vulnerable to many diseases as well as injuries, which explains the wide variety of treatments used. In some cases the variation may have reflected cultural (Galician or Bukovinian) or geographic (region or village) differences, which were not identified.

Skin conditions (Table 3) were the most commonly treated health problems and used a total of 319 different remedies. Infected wounds, boils, chapped skin, and bleeding cuts were the most common problems dealt with. Insect bites, fleas, and slivers were the least serious problems encountered, and were more an annoyance than a health threat.

> Sometimes when the children had a sore (bil) that would not heal, Mother covered it with some fresh cow manure and wrapped it on for a few hours. For a bad wound (rana), she left it on overnight. It really seemed to pull out the pus (hnii) and help the healing. She had heard older farmers talking about treating problem wounds in this way. — M. U. / Innisfree

Head-related conditions (Table 4) were the next most common health issues treated with traditional methods. Remedies focused on treating headaches, sore

TABLE 4    Variety of home treatments and materials used for head-related conditions

| Medical Condition | Treatments and Materials Used | Informant Use |
|---|---|---|
| Sore throat | 52 | 151 |
| Headache | 37 | 228 |
| Fever | 29 | 129 |
| Toothache | 24 | 83 |
| Earache | 20 | 77 |
| Eye problems | 19 | 63 |
| Lice (head) | 6 | 105 |
| **Total** | **187** | **836** |

TABLE 5    Variety of home treatments and materials used for gastrointestinal and liver conditions

| Medical Condition | Treatments and Materials Used | Informant Use |
|---|---|---|
| Abdominal pain | 52 | 231 |
| Constipation | 39 | 98 |
| Diarrhea | 34 | 104 |
| Parasites | 22 | 43 |
| Appetite (enhancement) | 13 | 61 |
| Poisoning (food) | 12 | 20 |
| Vomiting (induction) | 10 | 23 |
| Ulcers | 6 | 9 |
| Gallbladder problems | 5 | 7 |
| Liver problems | 2 | 2 |
| **Total** | **195** | **598** |

TABLE 6    Variety of home treatments and materials used for respiratory tract conditions

| Medical Condition | Treatments and Materials Used | Informant Use |
|---|---|---|
| Cold and flu | 55 | 302 |
| Nasal congestion | 29 | 45 |
| Shortness of breath (asthma) | 15 | 19 |
| Consumption (tuberculosis) | 4 | 4 |
| Croup (bronchitis) | 1 | 1 |
| **Total** | **104** | **371** |

throats, fevers, and head lice. Eye, ear, and tooth problems presented greater challenges and, when possible, would have been taken to a doctor for treatment.

> *My youngest daughter was playing in the grass* (trava) *and accidentally got a grass seed in her eye* (oko). *She began to scream* (krychaty) *in pain and was rubbing her eye. I pulled back the eyelid and with the tip of a cloth was able to remove the irritating seed.* — S. R. / Smoky Lake

Gastrointestinal problems (Table 5) were mainly expressed as abdominal pain, diarrhea, and constipation. Less frequently reported were problems related to ulcers, the gallbladder, and the liver. These conditions and organs were less likely to be treated with kitchen medicine, and usually required medical intervention. Constipation was not as much of a problem for the older generation, due to a diet rich in vegetables and because of the hard physical work of farm life. It may have been more of a problem for the young, who were fussier eaters, and it would certainly have been a greater problem in the winter season, when vegetables were less readily available.

Respiratory tract conditions (Table 6) that were commonly treated with home medicines included colds and the flu, as well as their associated nasal congestion. Consumption (tuberculosis) and croup (bronchitis) were less frequently reported, probably because they were less likely to be recognized as separate and distinct health conditions, and would not have responded well to home remedies.

Alcohol, primarily whisky, was used by adult Ukrainians as a preventative measure against catching a cold or flu. During the 1918–1919 Spanish influenza outbreak, homebrew and garlic were "medicines" much sought after in Ukrainian settlement communities — by Ukrainians and other Canadians alike.

General health concerns (Table 7) cover a range of the more behavioural and emotional conditions. Unspecified malaise ("not feeling well"), hangover, child fussiness, and sleeplessness were the most reported conditions treated. Adults knew the importance of staying healthy, because farm work did not provide the luxury of time off for rest and recuperation. Fatigue, nervousness, and poor health were problems less commonly dealt with using home remedies.

TABLE 7    Variety of home treatments and materials used for general health conditions

| Medical Condition | Treatments and Materials Used | Informant Use |
|---|---|---|
| Lack of well-being | 39 | 123 |
| Sleeplessness | 17 | 36 |
| Hangover | 12 | 43 |
| Fussiness / colic | 10 | 69 |
| Fatigue / run down | 9 | 14 |
| Nervousness / anxiety | 7 | 13 |
| Poor health / pain | 5 | 12 |
| **Total** | **139** | **310** |

TABLE 8    Variety of home treatments and materials used for musculoskeletal conditions

| Medical Condition | Treatments and Materials Used | Informant Use |
|---|---|---|
| Arthritis and rheumatism | 37 | 111 |
| Aches and pains | 33 | 154 |
| Swollen hands and feet | 12 | 18 |
| Abdominal strain | 5 | 12 |
| Chilling | 5 | 11 |
| Breaks and sprains* | 2 | 2 |
| **Total** | **94** | **308** |

*most of these types of injuries were treated by a bonesetter

TABLE 9    Variety of home treatments and materials used for circulatory and urinary conditions

| Medical Condition | Treatments and Materials Used | Informant Use |
|---|---|---|
| Kidney and bladder problems | 26 | 100 |
| Heart and blood problems | 26 | 87 |
| Dehydration | 2 | 4 |
| Hemorrhoids | 1 | 1 |
| **Total** | **55** | **192** |

Musculoskeletal problems (Table 8) were widespread, with aches and pains being the most common complaints recognized. Adults knew that aches and pains were an everyday feature of life and work. You simply had to bear them with as little discomfort as possible, because in most cases they simply required rest and relaxation as an immediate treatment and resolved themselves with time. In the old days no one complained about or discussed their pain, they just lived with and through it. Rheumatism and arthritis were the most common health issues for the elderly and were not only painful but crippling conditions. During these times, people did not understand the medical aspects of the different forms of arthritis and rheumatism and simply tried to alleviate their painful symptoms. In desperation, they tried and applied whatever brought relief from pain, even if it was only temporary. Chills, abdominal strains, and breaks and sprains were less often treated with home remedies but were more commonly treated by such folk healers as bonesetters and midwives. Broken bones and sprained limbs required special treatment, and bonesetters saved many a limb or digit that doctors might have otherwise amputated. Their work also prevented many settlers from living their lives in a crippled state.

Circulatory and urinary conditions (Table 9) can be serious health problems, with the former being life threatening. Heart and blood conditions would initially be treated with a variety of folk remedies, but in most cases would have then been treated by either a folk healer (bloodletting) or a doctor (medication or surgery). Urinary problems were seen as treatable with home remedies, which often resolved the condition.

Common diseases (Table 10) treated with home remedies were mainly childhood conditions such as chicken pox and measles. The adult (Type 2) form of diabetes, which is more manageable with dietary changes, was also treated with folk remedies. Cancer, diphtheria, and whooping cough were serious illnesses that required a doctor's treatment. Diphtheria, measles, mumps, and chicken pox were also contagious, and although attempts were made to keep the sick person away from others, it was difficult to do in large families with crowded living conditions.

Female health concerns (Table 11) showed the fewest informant responses and treatment forms, because it would be uncommon for a woman to discuss such things openly with a man. I sensed the discomfort in my informants when

TABLE 10    Variety of home treatments and materials used for common diseases

| Major Illness | Treatments and Materials Used | Informant Use |
|---|---|---|
| Chicken pox | 9 | 23 |
| Diabetes | 7 | 17 |
| Diphtheria | 3 | 3 |
| Measles | 3 | 13 |
| Cancer | 3 | 5 |
| Whooping cough | 1 | 1 |
| **Total** | **26** | **62** |

TABLE 11    Variety of home treatments and materials used for female conditions

| Medical Condition | Treatments and Materials Used | Informant Use |
|---|---|---|
| Menstrual cramps | 14 | 18 |
| Pregnancy | 10 | 14 |
| Birthing | 5 | 7 |
| **Total** | **29** | **39** |

I asked questions on this topic, and therefore the responses mostly focused on menstrual cramps and pregnancy issues. Specific health problems, such as yeast infections or other genital conditions, were never raised. The actual birthing process, and its complications, were handled by either a midwife (most often) or by a doctor (less often).

> Mother was a midwife and tried to help women who could not get pregnant. She would collect dry red onion skins and place these onto a plate of hot embers. The "barren" woman, wearing a long and loose-fitting gown or dress (suknia), would have to stand over the smouldering onion skins. The smoke rose up under her gown, over her body, and out through the collar area. She also had to inhale some of the escaping smoke (dym). This treatment was supposed to help her get pregnant (vahitna). — P. L. / Willingdon

Generally, people attempted to deal with the simpler and more treatable health problems by using folk remedies. Everyone's body and health are slightly different, and if one treatment did not work, another would be tried. Often it would be only a matter of time before the body's natural healing processes successfully dealt with the condition. Using a folk treatment may in many cases have had no more than a placebo effect, because the person believed they would get better from the treatment and ultimately did. In any community there would have been a wide range of treatments used, and people shared such knowledge freely with one another. In many cases, someone visiting a family was able to suggest a successful remedy for some health problem in the home. Older women, more experienced and knowledgeable in such matters, were most often the sources of such successful treatments. Additionally, specialized folk healers such as bonesetters, midwives, and spiritual healers were available to deal with more challenging and serious health issues. Doctors were initially used as a last resort, not only because of the difficulty in accessing them, but also because of the cost of such treatment.

> In the Old Country, a woman's leg (noha) became badly infected, and the doctors wanted to amputate it. She did not want to lose her leg, so she would not agree to the operation. A stranger, stopping by to beg for some bread, noticed her enormously swollen leg and said he knew a treatment that might save her leg. She was told to mix some lime, used for whitewashing buildings, with water (voda) and then to let the lime settle out. She was then to soak a towel (rushnyk) in the water above the settled lime, wrap the towel around the injured leg, and keep the leg covered with blankets overnight. She did this, and when she got up the next morning she was amazed to see that the swelling had gone down. Only sagging skin remained from the swelling, and in time the leg healed completely. — A. C. / Mundare

There was also a matter of treatment acceptance, and in the early days conventional medicine was viewed with a degree of distrust because of its heavy reliance on drugs and surgery. When I asked informants "what they did *(shcho vony robyly)*" for some specific health problem, the most common response was they "did whatever they knew *(robyly shcho znaly)*". Traditional home remedies were familiar, made use of available—and in most cases, natural—materials, were not invasive, were typically safe, were effective to some degree, and were inexpensive. In many ways, the Ukrainian bloc settlements were self-sufficient for most of their basic health care needs. Only when doctors and drugs became more locally available did the younger generation show a greater acceptance and dependence on them. Fear of ridicule and a sense of shame, not ineffectiveness, were the major reasons for the growing reluctance to use traditional Ukrainian home remedies and treatments.

# SEVEN

# Homestead Healing Resources

Over the centuries, in the Old Country, Ukrainian folk medicine had developed a rich heritage and tradition of simple but effective remedies and practices. These were readily transplanted throughout the regions of Ukrainian settlement in Canada and were supported by the presence, in the communities, of various traditional folk healers who provided more specialized physical and spiritual healing treatments (see chapter four).

Home-based healing was therefore widely practised and essential to survival on isolated homesteads. Kitchen medicine was often the difference between good health or illness and, in extreme cases, between life and death. Many a foot or finger was saved from amputation by the successful use of a home remedy using simple ingredients. Children were often nursed back to health with a simple concoction of household materials that not only provided relief from discomfort but also healed the problem. The kitchen was not only the family's "hospital," it was also its "drugstore," demonstrating the settlers' near total self-reliance.

*My husband* (cholovik), *wearing only a shirt, had been working outside on a rainy and windy day and got very chilled* (zastudyvsia). *He came into the house* (khata) *and sat down by the hot stove to warm up. After laying down to rest, he got up but felt both dizzy and chilled. A neighbour* (susid), *who once suffered the same condition, suggested a treatment that used alcohol, a bar of store-bought wash soap, and some grassy herbs. I gathered hay and herbs from the forest nearby and boiled these in a large pot. I strained the liquid into a washtub and then added some more hot water. My husband sat over the tub* (baliia), *covered*

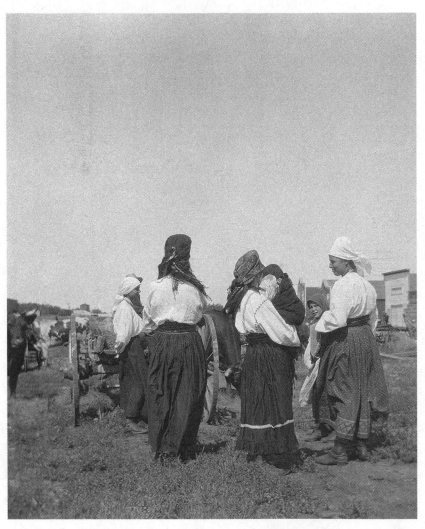

Women socialized and helped one another whenever they got together. [PAM N11586]

*himself with a heavy bedsheet, and steamed himself as long as he could bear the heat. He then lay down on a bench (lavka), and I rubbed his body thoroughly with the alcohol and soap. He then went to bed (lizhko), well covered with sheets and blankets, to sweat some more. We repeated this treatment once again, and he recovered completely.* — K. N. / Smoky Lake

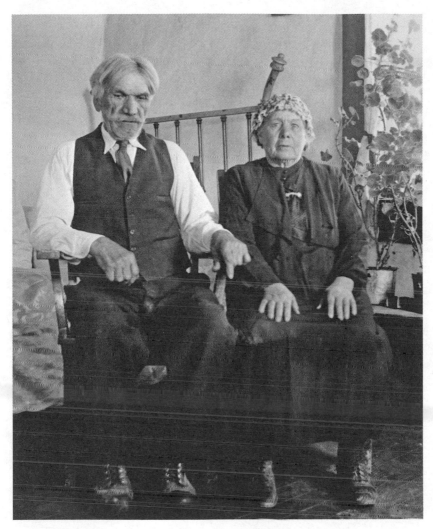

Grandfather and grandmother were important family resources. [PAM N9174]

Folk healing traditions relied heavily on women and their sensitive, caring, and compassionate nature. A family's health and well-being was typically the responsibility of the mother, often supplemented with the expertise of a live-in grandmother or an elderly female neighbour. In times of desperate need, community resources could be drawn upon for advice, essential healing preparations, or specialized assistance. The success of the early Ukrainian settlers was therefore based on a combination of self-reliance and community outreach.

*My mother was carrying a pot of hot water* (hariacha voda) *to the table and some of it splashed on my bare feet. The burned skin* (shkira) *blistered, and my mother did not know what to do for me. An older woman visiting us told her to go to the slough and collect a frog's "nest" [egg mass?]. The material was wet and slimy, but it did help the blisters to heal well.* — M. S. / Vegreville

Older men were also an important community healing resource, because many of them would have been exposed to paramedical training during their compulsory service in the Austro-Hungarian army. Such knowledge would have served them well in dealing with more serious wounds and bone injuries. Those with interest and practical experience in naturopathic healing would have been able to provide such services as bloodletting, cupping, and the application of leeches. Some brought from the Old Country specialized splint boards, bandages, skin laceration knives, and suction cups for their treatments.

Traditional home remedies were generally quite effective for simple everyday or seasonal health problems. For other health conditions, such as major diseases, they were less effective and at best provided the sick person with only a small degree of comfort and relief. Even so, this was especially important to children, who would not know what was happening to them and who would have much lower tolerance to pain and discomfort. A strong religious faith, characteristic of the Ukrainian settlers, also provided comfort and relief in their suffering. For serious illness, belief in divine intervention and healing would have been the last resort to draw upon. Collectively, these various direct and indirect interventions helped the sick person believe in a cure and get better. Nevertheless, this did not occur without much collective worry and suffering. In some cases, even after exhausting all possible folk treatments, the result was tragic—as it was for the many women and babies who died during childbirth.

Healing materials used to treat a specific condition could vary greatly from household to household because of regional differences in their development

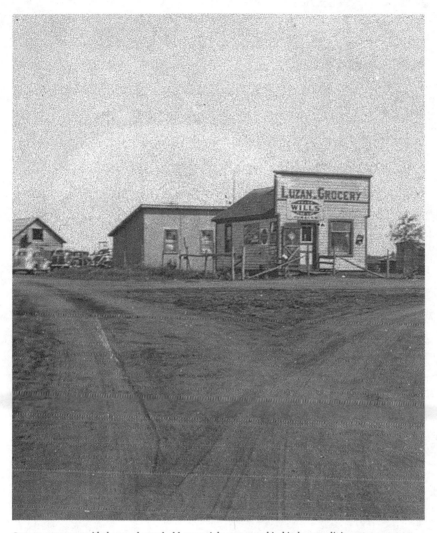

Country stores provided many household essentials, some used in kitchen medicines. [PAA UV65]

and use. Most remedies used only a single ingredient, such as cranberry juice for a cold and cough. But other treatments might involve a combination of a few simple ingredients, such as garlic and warm milk, for the same condition. Farm, store-bought, and household products were the main ingredients of most home remedies. These materials were always available, relatively safe to

TABLE 12    Treatment Value of domesticated and native plant-based products used in home remedies

| Product | Treatment Value | Major Application(s) |
|---|---|---|
| a) solids: | | |
| Bread* | 79 | boils / cuts / infections / cold and flu / puncture wounds |
| Flour* | 74 | cuts / chest congestion / infections / boils |
| Sauerkraut | 37 | constipation / intestinal worms / frozen skin / tonic |
| Pickles | 7 | hangover / intestinal worms / pregnancy |
| b) liquids: | | |
| Homebrew* | 306 | lack of appetite / cold and flu / internal pain / toothache / sore throat / sleeplessness / tonic / rheumatism / muscle pain / burns / skin conditions / cuts / inflamed tonsils / nervousness / diarrhea |
| Pickle juice | 107 | internal pain / hangover / tonic / lack of appetite / intestinal worms / inducement of vomiting |
| Sauerkraut juice | 107 | internal pain / hangover / constipation / tonic / lack of appetite / thirst / ulcers |
| Vegetable oil | 44 | earache / burns / skin conditions |
| Fruit juice | 14 | cold and flu / tonic |

* often used in combination with other materials

use, and easily applied. Garden vegetables, herbs, and wild plants, which were typically dried or stored for winter use, were also important healing materials. Animal products, such as fats, were also readily available and were a major component of many healing preparations. Alcohol, especially locally made medicinal moonshine, was not only a curative material by itself but was also used in combination with other materials, especially in tinctures and other folk healing preparations.

> In our family, animal products were also used as medicine. Boiled pigeon (holub) meat was considered to be a very healthy food and was given to anyone who was weak or in poor health. Goat's milk (moloko vid kozy) was also considered healthy and was used for someone, especially a child, who was coughing, run down, or in poor health. Children seemed to recover (povertaty) much faster when they were given these to eat and drink. — C. O. / Edmonton

TABLE 13    Treatment Value of purchased plant-based products used in home remedies

| Product | Treatment Value | Major Application(s) |
| --- | --- | --- |
| a) *solids:* | | |
| Lemon* | 71 | cold and flu / sore throat / fever / nasal congestion / urinary problems / gallstones |
| Sugar* | 38 | eye problems / cold and flu / intestinal worms |
| Coffee | 18 | diarrhea / hangover |
| Tobacco | 15 | toothache |
| Tea | 12 | diarrhea / eye conditions / sore throat |
| Cornstarch | 10 | diaper rash |
| Fruit (whole) | 9 | constipation / internal pain |
| Snuff | 5 | nasal congestion |
| Barley (pearl) | 3 | diarrhea |
| Rice | 2 | diarrhea |
| Yeast | ** | boils |
| b) *spices:* | | |
| Mustard (dry)* | 44 | chest congestion / inducement of vomiting / sore throat |
| Black pepper* | 37 | internal pain / diarrhea / earache / cold and flu / toothache |
| Ginger | 14 | internal pain / cold and flu / menstrual cramps |
| Caraway seeds | 12 | internal pain |
| Cayenne pepper | 8 | cold and flu / nasal congestion / sore throat / breathing problems |
| Spices (various) | 5 | toothache / lack of appetite / internal pain |
| Cinnamon | 5 | pregnancy / diarrhea / intestinal worms |
| Anise | 4 | constipation |
| Senna | 3 | diarrhea / internal pain |
| Incense | 1 | chapped skin |
| Chili pepper | 1 | muscle aches |
| c) *liquids:* | | |
| Vinegar* | 171 | headache / fever / cold and flu / cuts / head lice / toothache / rheumatism |
| Molasses* | 11 | constipation / tonic |
| Wine | 7 | lack of appetite / tonic |
| Olive oil | 6 | earache |
| Vanilla | 5 | toothache / constipation |

* often used in combination with other materials
** TV less than 1

## HOUSEHOLD MATERIALS

Nutritious meals made with fresh ingredients contributed greatly to keeping people healthy, reducing illness, and helping the sick regain their health. A woman's careful management of her garden and household pantry ensured that each home had a constant inventory of healthy foods, many of which could also be used as ingredients in home remedies (Table 12). Those that were not kept on hand or that ran out were easily obtained from a neighbour. Flour, bread, whisky, and pickle juice were major healing ingredients. Whisky, as a healing agent, was extremely important in traditional Ukrainian folk medicine, but its legal availability during Prohibition was highly regulated by the government, and it could be purchased only with a doctor's prescription. Homebrew, although illegal to make or possess, became a major medical resource for many home remedies. Interestingly, kitchen-based ingredients served to treat a wide range of conditions and often overlapped in the problems they were used to treat.

Store-bought plant-based products (Table 13) were also important kitchen medicines. Lemons and sugar, as well as mustard, pepper, and vinegar, were important ingredients. These were mainly used for treating digestive problems and conditions associated with the head and chest.

Fresh or preserved (dried) fruits and vegetables were also important healing agents. Potatoes, onions, garlic, raspberries, strawberries, and herbs such as chamomile, parsley, mint, and chrysanthemum were widely used in various remedies. Many of the settlers, uncertain of which plants would be available in Canada, brought seeds or cuttings of medicinal plants for their gardens. Native plants, such as cranberries and puffballs, were prized healing materials. They were collected whenever possible and dried for use throughout the year. They were always available for someone's use in other households in the community.

> *I was working on a threshing gang, and we went to a new farm to thresh their grain* (zerno). *Somehow the food got bad and we all got sick* (slabi) *from food poisoning. One of the hired men, who had been a brewer in the Old Country, told my brother to go into town* (misto) *and buy a bottle of whisky and some powdered ginger. Each sick person was given a shot of whisky and a teaspoon of ginger. They all got better.* — D. O. / Vegreville

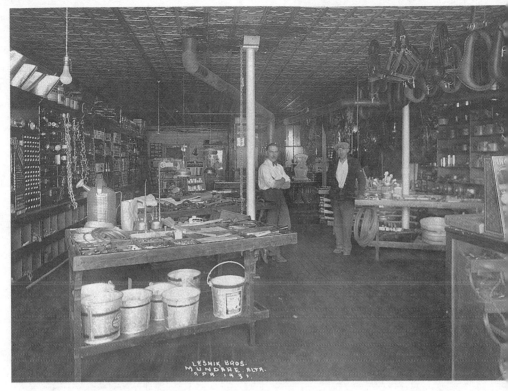

Farm supplies were also important sources of healing materials. [PAA UV019]

## FARM MATERIALS

Farm materials (Table 14) such as kerosene and axle grease were also effective healing agents, especially kerosene, which was used for both external and internal applications. Its main value was in controlling head lice, but it was also used to eliminate intestinal parasites. Axle grease, considered more potent if it had been already used on equipment, was used for skin conditions.

Soil, often simply called dirt, was also used as a healing agent. Clay, either the yellow or blue type, was dug up, dried, sieved, and saved in a paper bag for use on burns and a baby's irritated skin. Soil, if no other material was available, could also be applied and wrapped onto a bleeding wound. Soil fungi and microbes would have been the agents responsible for helping the wound to heal.

TABLE 14   Treatment Value of farm materials used in home healing practices

| Product | Treatment Value | Major Application(s) |
|---|---|---|
| Kerosene | 120 | head lice / intestinal worms / chest congestion / frozen skin / ringworm / toothache |
| Axle grease | 15 | ringworm / wounds |
| Machine oil | 7 | earache / burns / ringworm |
| Soap | 3 | constipation / head lice |
| Turpentine | 3 | nasal congestion / chest congestion |
| Gasoline | 1 | boils |
| Pine oil | ** | croup |
| Flax seed oil | ** | constipation |

* used in combination with other materials
** TV less than 1


TABLE 15   Treatment Value of purchased chemicals used in home healing practices

| Product | Treatment Value | Major Application(s) |
|---|---|---|
| Salt* | 93 | puncture wounds / sore throat / cuts / toothache / muscle pain |
| Baking soda* | 48 | burns / chicken pox / fever / diaper rash / internal pain |
| Sulphur* | 49 | skin conditions / boils / ringworm / intestinal worms |
| Epsom salts | 16 | puncture wounds |
| Blue stone (copper sulphate) | 8 | ringworm / toothache / skin conditions / eye conditions |
| Cream of tartar | 4 | urinary problems / infections |
| Lye | 1 | warts |
| Nitric acid | 1 | warts |
| Boric acid | 1 | eye conditions |
| Chalk | ** | warts |
| Rennin | ** | diarrhea |
| Glycerine | ** | earache |

* used in combination with other materials
** TV less than 1

*There was no baby powder or salve in the Old Days. When she needed something like that, Mother would take a shovel and dig up some yellow clay* (zhovta hlyna). *She dried it out and crumbled it up in a handkerchief, which she tied off to make a cloth bag. Shaking this "bag"* (mishok) *produced a fine powder that could be used to cover a baby's bottom and armpits. This prevented moist heat rash from forming and irritating the baby.* — N. S. / Viking


## CHEMICALS

Store-bought chemicals (Table 15) such as salt, baking soda, and sulphur were an important component of a wide variety of home medicines. They were typically used to deal with wounds or skin problems. Table salt and Epsom salts, dissolved in hot water, were very effective in cleaning open wounds, especially ones due to a puncture of the skin. Sulphur mixed in animal fat made an effective salve for skin rashes. Acidic and caustic materials were rarely used, and only to "burn" out warts.


## ANIMAL PRODUCTS

Animal products used in healing applications were primarily derived from processed (Table 16) or unprocessed (Tables 17 and 18) materials from domesticated farm animals. These were mainly used for treating various skin conditions, because they not only possessed healing properties but also kept the skin soft and pliable. Honey and dairy products were important processed ingredients, while milk, eggs, and fats were important unprocessed healing materials. Milk was especially important in home remedies for respiratory and digestive problems.

Fresh cow manure was commonly used on infected wounds that were not healing. Although an animal waste product, manure was full of undigested plant matter. This, plus its microbial components, would have had antibiotic-like qualities. Cow manure poultices were either the initial treatment for a deep wound or the final treatment for one that was festering and not healing well.

TABLE 16    Treatment Value of processed farm animal products used in home remedies

| Product | Treatment Value | Major Application(s) |
|---|---|---|
| Honey* | 99 | cold and flu / sore throat / sleeplessness / boils |
| Cream (sweet) | 96 | chapped skin / skin conditions / burns / diaper rash / frozen skin / ringworm |
| Butter* | 87 | cold and flu / chapped skin / burns / skin conditions / diaper rash / sore throat / sleeplessness / constipation |
| Cheese whey | 37 | infections / puncture wounds / bone injuries / tonic |
| Chicken soup | 10 | cold and flu |
| Buttermilk | 5 | chapped skin / skin rash / internal pain |
| Cottage cheese | 1 | tonic |
| Cream (sour) | ** | chapped skin |

* used in combination with other materials
** TV less than 1


TABLE 17    Treatment Value of unprocessed farm animal products used in home remedies

| Product | Treatment Value | Major Application(s) |
|---|---|---|
| Cow's milk* (fresh) | 278 | cold and flu / boils / infections / sore throat / diarrhea / cuts / sleeplessness / chest congestion / puncture wounds / constipation / poisoning |
| Eggs* (whole***/ boiled) | 68 | burns / diarrhea / skin conditions / cold and flu / infections |
| Cow's milk (sour) | 59 | poisoning / inducement of vomiting / hangover / fever / puncture wounds |
| Manure (cow*** or horse) | 14 | infections / boils / ringworm |
| Goat's milk | 5 | tonic / allergies / chest pain |
| Horse hair | 3 | warts |
| Pig's gallbladder | 3 | poisoning / infections |
| Feathers (duck or goose) | 3 | nasal congestion / diphtheria |
| Mare's milk | ** | measles |
| Pigeon blood | ** | warts |
| Pigeon meat | ** | tonic |
| Sheep's brain | ** | boils |

* used in combination with other materials
** TV less than 1
*** most commonly used

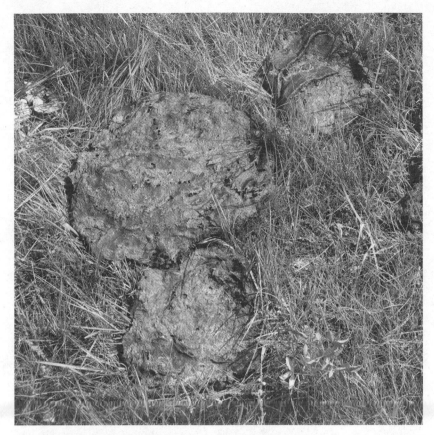

Fresh cow manure was used to help heal wounds. [M. MUCZ]

*Whenever Father (Batko) had a bad cut or bruise, where the skin was broken, he would treat it to prevent infection. He took fresh cow manure, which seemed to have some healing materials in it. He smeared the manure on the injury and left it on for a while or sometimes even wrapped it on with a cloth. It was really helpful in getting the wound to heal.* — L. K. / Star

Native animal products (Table 19) used for home healing were readily available from the surrounding bush and water bodies. Leeches were commonly used for removing "bad" blood. Wild animal fats were used to treat skin problems.

TABLE 18    Treatment Value of unprocessed farm animal fats and oils used in home remedies

| Product | Treatment Value | Major Application(s) |
|---|---|---|
| Pork fat | 130 | chapped skin / chest congestion / burns / open cuts / cold and flu / diaper rash / boils / chicken pox |
| Goose fat* | 126 | chapped skin / chest congestion / cold and flu / skin conditions / burns |
| Chicken fat | 11 | chapped skin / infections / diaper rash |
| Beef tallow | 5 | muscle aches / birthing / earache |
| Sheep fat | 4 | chapped skin / burns |
| Sheep wool lanolin | 3 | frozen skin / warts |
| Dog fat | ** | consumption (tuberculosis) |

* used in combination with other materials
** TV less than 1


TABLE 19    Treatment Value factors of natural (wild) animal materials used in home remedies

| Product | Treatment Value | Major Application(s) |
|---|---|---|
| Leeches | 59 | muscle aches and pains / "bad" blood / rheumatism / swelling / chilled body / headache |
| Bear fat* | 8 | rheumatism / skin conditions / chapped skin / frozen skin |
| Beeswax | 5 | skin conditions / chapped skin |
| Badger fat* | 5 | chapped skin / cold and flu / cuts |
| Skunk fat* | ** | infections |
| Bee venom | ** | arthritis and rheumatism |

* used when available
** TV less than 1


# PLANT MATERIALS

Globally, especially in the developing world, plant-based (herbal) traditional medicine continues to be more popular than conventional medicine. Most herb-based treatments are highly effective in providing relief, with minimal side effects, for a wide range of health problems. A large number of healing plants are weedy species and therefore are common in areas with high human activity. Weeds, mainly annual plants, develop an effective variety of self-defence chemicals (secondary metabolites) for protection against insect and animal feeding. These same compounds provide healing components in home remedies. Domesticated plants are also known to have healing properties, and Ukrainian folk remedies use both groups of plants as healing agents.

*I was sixteen years old when I froze my foot* (stopa) *so badly that I could not even take my shoe* (cherevyk) *off. My mother finally did get my foot out, but did not know what to do. The next morning, seeing that my foot was swollen and badly blistered, she remembered an Old Country home remedy that used peas* (horokh). *She soaked some dry peas, and when they were soft, she mashed them up. She placed the pea mash on my foot, and wrapped it on. She changed the pea poultice* (pryparka) *daily, and in a week the blistering was all gone. The skin also began healing, and in five weeks my foot was well enough for me to put my shoe on again.* — H. J. / Vegreville

Herbs are generally described as non-woody plants with medicinal or food uses. If they were not grown in the garden or a separate medicinal herb garden, then such healing materials were gathered from the wild. Collection was generally done in the late morning, when plants were free of dew but not yet wilted from the sun's heat. Medicinally effective parts, such as flowers, leaves, or roots, were collected only from healthy, intact plants. Plant parts had different levels of medicinal effectiveness during their life cycle. Stems and leaves were best before or during the blooming period; flowers during early to mid-bloom; roots in the fall or early spring, when their stored reserves were highest; seeds and fruits when ripe but before they had been released; buds in early spring, when they were still swollen and not yet green; and bark in the spring, from young (three- to four-year-old) branches.

Harvested non-woody plant materials were rinsed free of dirt and debris, while woody tissues (roots, bark, twigs, stems) were chopped up into smaller pieces, prior to drying. All materials were always dried thoroughly to ensure that they did not get mouldy and lose medicinal potency. Plants with non-volatile materials were air dried quickly in the sun, but those with volatile oils, which were highly aromatic, were dried more slowly in a well-ventilated room. The dry parts were then stored in paper or cloth bags or in jars covered with paper. Often whole plants were simply tied together and hung upside down, inside the house, along the edge of the ceiling. If no dried plant materials were available, or if their supply had run out, sorting through stored hay might yield bits and pieces of desired species. Neighbours could also be asked to share their supply of such plants, and they did so willingly, knowing that they might have similar needs in the future.

Dried plant materials were often used in making teas or infusions (see description in chapter nine). These were easily and quickly prepared for use by older children and adults. Younger children found such teas too bitter to drink and needed to have them sweetened with sugar or honey. Herbal preparations not only provided a variety of healing agents, but were also a source of much-needed minerals and vitamins.

> *I gathered a lot of nettle* (kropyva) *and dried it. When I needed to use it,*
> *I soaked it in water and then boiled it a bit. I strained the liquid and drank it,*
> *a half a cup at a time, three times a day. The old people* (stari liudy) *said that*
> *it was good for treating arthritis and rheumatism, as well as many stomach*
> (shlunok) *problems.* — M. M. / Vegreville

Traditional Ukrainian medicine made extensive use of both native (wild) and cultivated species (Table 20). These healing plants were readily found in the meadows and forests surrounding villages and farms, and were preserved (dried) for later use. Many of the plants the settlers would have known as native species in the Old Country were present in Canada as accidentally introduced weed species.

Although fresh plant material was preferred in preparing home remedies, dried plants were easier to use throughout the year. Root vegetables were also always available, and many of these were used as home healing agents. Often only one plant was used in a remedy, or at the most no more than three. The simplicity of Ukrainian folk medicine's plant use contrasts with the more complex use of plants in Traditional Chinese Medicine, where herbal preparations consist of six to twelve different plant species.

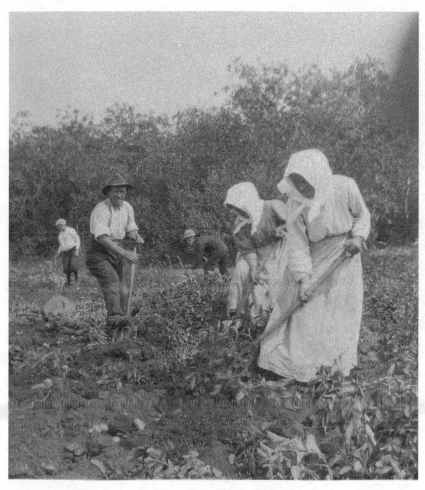

The garden's importance meant that everyone worked in it. [PAM N9637]

Either the entire plant was prepared, or only parts, such as the flowers, leaves, or roots. Plant tissues contain a diversity of chemical constituents and can be used to treat a wide range of health problems. Plants are therefore the most natural and safe holistic chemical treatment for most basic human illnesses, and time and again they are shown to be highly effective. Their major drawback is that they are not as fast-acting as drug preparations, but their advantage is that they have fewer potentially severe side effects.

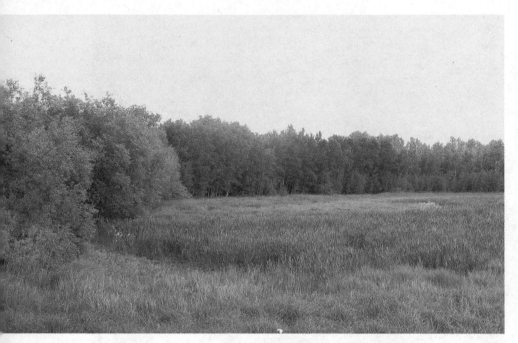

Local forests, grasslands, and wetlands supplied native medicinal plants. [M. MUCZ]

## Native Plants

Natalia Osadcha-Janata, in her 1952 publication *Herbs Used in Ukrainian Folk Medicine* (see Selected Readings), recorded 646 plant species from the Ukrainian flora as being used in regional folk remedies. Of these, 50 to 60 per cent are herbs. Of the eighty-nine species described in detail, a number of them were used in remedies for various diseases. My study revealed similar widespread use of the same species in a number of treatments, but I recorded only forty-six native (wild) species that Ukrainian settlers in Canada used for medicinal purposes (Appendix II). Two thirds of these are herbaceous or non-woody species, a number similar to Osadcha-Janata's findings. The most widely used healing plants identified in this study (Table 20) were non-woody species such as colts-foot, wormwood, plantain, nettle, yarrow, strawberry, dandelion, and burdock; shrubs such as cranberry, raspberry, and rose; medicinally useful trees such as linden, conifers (spruce and pine), and birch; and fungal puffballs.

| TABLE 20 | Native and domesticated plants commonly used in home remedies |
|---|---|
| Fungus | puffball, birch fungus |
| Trees | linden, paper birch, spruce, pine |
| Shrubs | blueberry, cranberry, raspberry, juniper, rose |
| Weeds | plantain, dandelion, yarrow, nettle, burdock, coltsfoot, wormwood |
| Ornamental | chrysanthemum / costmary, aloe |
| Vegetable / Crop | flax, oats, tobacco, carrot, cabbage, potato, parsnip, beets, hemp, poppy, strawberry |
| Herbs / Spices | lovage, mint, chamomile, garlic, parsley, lemon, mustard, onion, horseradish, ginger, cinnamon, black pepper, feverfew, caraway, costmary |

*Wormwood* (polyn) *is good for your health, and you should drink its tea* (chai) *twice a week. It does two things for you: it thins out your blood* (krov) *if it is too thick, and it can produce more blood if the levels are too low. I knew a man who looked run down and pale in appearance, so I gave him some wormwood to try. He was not sure if he would use it, but once he did, he felt much better, and his skin colour had a healthier appearance. He was very grateful for my help in recovering his health, because the doctors had not been able to help him.* — A. B. / Camrose

A wide range of health problems were treated with native plant species (Table 21). Coltsfoot and plantain were used for various external applications, and wormwood was a major treatment for internal digestive upset. Stinging nettle, often used directly, was applied to painful arthritic areas for temporary relief. Yarrow was used for a variety of internal and external applications. Raspberry, cranberry, and blueberry were used for a diversity of internal health problems, but primarily pregnancy, colds and flu, and diabetes, respectively. Spruce, pine, and birch were used for skin problems, and linden flowers for colds and flu symptoms.

*My brother was teasing a dog* (pes), *and it bit him on the leg. The wound turned blue and became infected. Mother gathered up some young birch* (bereza) *twigs and boiled them for a long time. She soaked the leg in the hot solution and then wrapped coltsfoot leaves on the wound. This treatment healed up the wound completely, and he did not have to go to the doctor.* — C. O. / Edmonton

TABLE 21    Treatment Value of native plants used in home remedies

| Plant | Treatment Value | Major Application(s) |
|---|---|---|
| a) *fungi:* | | |
| Puffball | 39 | cuts / infections / puncture woulds / burns |
| Birch fungus | 11 | infections / wounds |
| b) *spore-bearing plants:* | | |
| Common horsetail | 1 | urinary problems |
| c) *broad-leaved plants:* | | |
| Arrow-leaved coltsfoot | 117 | infections / cuts / boils / puncture wounds / burns / swelling |
| Strawberry | 32 | diarrhea / fever / tonic / cold and flu / internal pain |
| Seneca root | 6 | tonic |
| Violet | 2 | infections / cold and flu · |
| Three-flowered avens | 1 | circulatory problems |
| Cow Parsnip | 1 | boils |
| Lily of the valley | 1 | breathing problems |
| d) *weeds:* | | |
| Wormwood | 299 | internal pain / intestinal worms / diabetes / urinary problems / lack of appetite / rheumatism / diarrhea / cancer / headache / swelling / menstrual pain / poisoning |
| Stinging nettle | 108 | rheumatism / muscle pain / cold and flu / headache / swelling / internal pain / tonic / wounds / swelling |
| Broad-leaved plantain | 89 | infections / boils / cuts / puncture wounds / skin conditions |
| Yarrow | 74 | urinary problems / cuts / internal pain / circulatory problems / diabetes / menstrual pain |
| Common dandelion | 26 | tonic / warts / urinary problems / cold and flu |
| Common burdock | 17 | internal pain |
| Sow thistle | 6 | warts |
| Common tansy | 3 | infections / intestinal worms |
| Canada thistle | 3 | cold and flu / swelling |
| Lamb's quarters | 3 | wounds / constipation |
| Black Henbane | 2 | toothache |
| Common mullein | 1 | toothache |

TABLE 21   Treatment Value of native plants used in home remedies (cont.)

| Plant | Treatment Value | Major Application(s) |
|---|---|---|
| Pineapple weed | 1 | internal pain |
| Dock | 1 | internal pain |
| e) grasses: | | |
| Couch grass | 3 | rheumatism / tonic |
| Cattail | 1 | cuts |
| f) shrubs: | | |
| Raspberry | 87 | tonic / cold and flu / fever / internal pain / pregnancy / eye conditions |
| Cranberry (highbush and lowbush) | 75 | cold and flu / urinary problems / fever / sore throat / general illness / tonic |
| Rose | 65 | tonic / cold and flu / constipation / chilling / circulatory problems |
| Blueberry | 25 | diarrhea / internal pain / constipation / diabetes |
| Creeping juniper | 12 | tonic |
| Willow | 9 | internal pain |
| Chokecherry | 3 | cold and flu / diarrhea |
| Currant | 3 | cold and flu / diarrhea |
| Round-leaved hawthorn | 3 | rheumatism / circulatory problems |
| Pin cherry | 3 | nasal congestion / sore throat |
| Common bearberry | 1 | urinary problems |
| g) trees: | | |
| Spruce and pine | 42 | skin conditions / internal pain |
| Linden | 37 | cold and flu / tonic |
| Paper birch | 18 | swelling / wounds |
| Balsam poplar | 8 | cuts / burns / skin conditions / boils |
| Trembling aspen | 1 | boils |

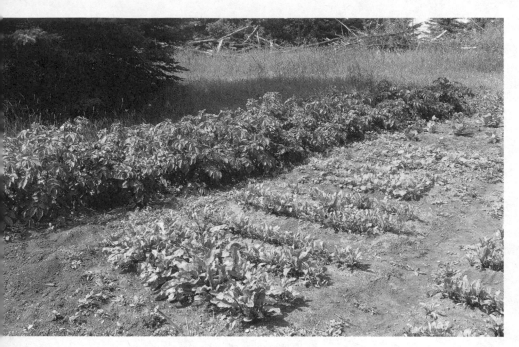

Gardens provided many cultivated healing plants. [M. MUCZ]

Antibiotics had not yet been discovered during the settlement period, but various fungal materials served similar purposes. Folk medicine had long recognized, dating back to the ancient Egyptians, the value of fungal moulds in treating wounds. Ukrainian settlers collected ripe puffballs for this purpose and stored reserves for use throughout the year. Bleeding or infected wounds to which puffball spores were applied healed more quickly. When these were unavailable, mouldy bread or mould growing on the top of spoiled beet soup *(borshch)* was applied to infected wounds and produced similar results.

> *My husband was working on a threshing machine and caught some fingers in its belt. The crushed fingers bled badly, and the man working with him quickly collected some ripe puffballs* (porkhavka)*. The bleeding stopped when the crushed fingers were placed, a few times, into the powdery centres of the puffballs. The spores also helped the fingers to heal well.* — E. L. / Two Hills

## Cultivated Plants

This study identified thirty-three garden (Appendix III) and eight crop (Appendix IV) species that were used in traditional healing remedies (Table 20). Potatoes, cabbage, and beets were the most commonly used vegetables; garlic, onion, chamomile, parsley, horseradish, mint, costmary, and feverfew were important herbs. Poppies and tobacco were common garden plants used in home remedies. A cactus, probably aloe, was the only houseplant described as being used for healing purposes. Of the field crops, flax, oats, and hemp were the most important.

> *My brother* (brat) *had a terrible eczema-like skin rash, and Mother cleared it up with her own homemade oil* (oliia). *It was made by slowly heating hemp seeds. The oil was extremely dark in colour and was called "soil oil"* (zemliana oliia). *It was a very fast-acting oil and cleared the rash up.* — A. C. / Smoky Lake

Much like the native species, garden and crop species were used for a variety of health conditions (Tables 22 and 23). Potatoes were used for treating headaches and skin conditions, while cabbage was used for headaches and as an internal remedy. Beets were used in treating internal conditions, primarily those associated with the circulatory system. Garlic, chamomile, and onions had a wide diversity of applications of primarily an internal nature. Parsley was primarily used for treating urinary problems, and horseradish for congestion and muscle pain. Mint, costmary, and feverfew were typically used to relieve pain symptoms. Poppy and tobacco were used as a sedative and toothache suppressant respectively. Aloe's gelatinous pulp was important in treating various skin conditions.

> *I froze my toe* (palets na nozi) *so badly that I developed a fever and could not sleep* (spaty). *Mother went to the sauerkraut barrel and brought back a fermented cabbage leaf* (lystok vid kapusty), *which she wrapped around the injured toe. I fell asleep easily, and by the next morning I only had to soak the toe in some warm water, but the toe was fine.* — M. D. / Vegreville

TABLE 22    Treatment Value of domesticated (garden, yard, and household) plants used
in home healing practices

| Plant | Treatment Value | Major Application(s) |
|---|---|---|
| *a) vegetables:* | | |
| Potato | 75 | headache / fever / infections / boils / rheumatism / burns |
| Cabbage | 68 | headache / fever / rheumatism / constipation / ulcers |
| Beets | 50 | circulatory problems / cold and flu / headache / urinary problems / constipation |
| Carrot | 11 | eye conditions |
| Rhubarb | 9 | circulatory problems |
| Radish | 4 | cold and flu |
| Beans | 3 | constipation / skin conditions |
| Turnip | 3 | urinary problems / internal pain |
| Peas | 3 | frozen skin / circulatory problems |
| Asparagus | 1 | urinary problems |
| Celery (seed) | 1 | intestinal worms |
| *b) herbs:* | | |
| Garlic* | 303 | cold and flu / chest congestion / circulatory problems / lack of appetite / fever / fatigue / sore throat / headache / toothache / rheumatism / intestinal worms / internal pain / tonic / nasal congestion |
| Chamomile | 225 | internal pain / headache / fever / cold and flu / colic / diarrhea / nervousness / pregnancy / sleeplessness / urinary problems / general illness / birthing / sore throat |
| Onion* | 184 | boils / cold and flu / infections / chest congestion / wounds / puncture wounds / fever / sore throat / burns / sleeplessness / internal pain / circulatory problems |
| Parsley | 96 | urinary problems / fever / cold and flu / circulatory problems / chest congestion / nasal congestion / internal pain |
| Horseradish | 88 | puncture wounds / cold and flu / chest congestion / muscle pain / internal pain / headache |
| Mint | 70 | internal pain / cold and flu / tonic / pregnancy |
| Costmary / Chrysanthemum | 61 | internal pain / general illness / infections |
| Feverfew | 40 | internal pain / chest congestion / constipation |
| Parsnip | 21 | urinary problems |
| Basil (seed*** / foliage) | 14 | eye problems |
| Lovage | 10 | infections / puncture wounds |

| Plant | Treatment Value | Major Application(s) |
|---|---|---|
| Comfrey | 4 | rheumatism |
| Thyme | 4 | internal pain |
| Dill | 2 | breathing problems |
| Sage | 1 | cold and flu |
| *c) garden / ornamentals:* | | |
| Poppy | 47 | sedative / toothache |
| Tobacco | 16 | toothache |
| Fern | 3 | rheumatism / burns |
| Bachelor button | 3 | menstrual pain / internal pain |
| Monkshood | 1 | sedative |
| Sweet william | 1 | eye problems |
| *d) houseplants:* | | |
| Cactus (aloe) | 21 | wounds / infections / burns |

\* used in combination with other materials
\*\* most used portion

TABLE 23   Treatment Value of field crop plants used in home remedies

| Plant | Treatment Value | Major Application(s) |
|---|---|---|
| Flax | 87 | constipation / boils / infections / internal pain / skin conditions |
| Oats | 39 | sore throat / muscle pain / rheumatism / headache |
| Hemp | 26 | skin conditions / sleeplessness / burns / cold and flu |
| Barley | 5 | diarrhea |
| Alfalfa | 1 | rheumatism |
| Buckwheat | 1 | fever |
| Clover | 1 | cold and flu |
| Rye | 1 | infections |

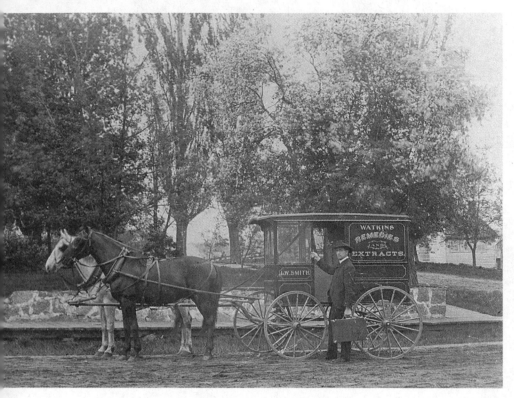

Travelling salesmen provided a variety of household and health care products.

## PATENT MEDICINES

In cities and larger towns, general stores and drugstores carried patent medicines and other prepared medicinal products. People in rural areas often purchased such items through catalogue orders (Eaton's in Winnipeg) or from travelling salesmen (Watkins, Rawleigh). These salesmen came through settlement areas, two or more times a year, by horse-drawn buggy or wagon and offered a range of household and farm products. In later times of greater prosperity, each rural area had its own local sales representative, and these products became available throughout the year. These representatives, typically male in the early years, not only sold various products, they also brought news of developments in products and practices from the "outside world." They provided helpful treatment

TABLE 24   Treatment Value of patent medicines used in home healing practices

| Product | Treatment Value | Major Application(s) |
|---|---|---|
| Ointments and salves* | 267 | muscle aches and pains / rheumatism / chest congestion / sore throat / skin conditions / internal pain / burns / toothache / nasal congestion / wounds |
| Vaseline | 48 | chapped skin / skin conditions / diaper rash / burns |
| Iodine | 21 | cuts / toothache / intestinal worms |
| Camphor oil | 13 | earache / nasal congestion / sleeplessness |
| Hoffmann's Drops | 11 | cold and flu / nasal congestion |
| Cod liver oil | 5 | chapped skin / constipation / internal pain |
| Vicks ointment | 4 | nasal congestion |
| Mint oil | 3 | diarrhea |
| Aspirin | 3 | menstrual cramps / warts |
| Carbolic salve | 3 | burns / diaper rash |
| Creoline ointment | 2 | puncture wounds / ringworm |
| Castor oil | 2 | constipation |
| Kidney pills | ** | urinary problems |
| Cough syrup | ** | sore throat |
| Zinc ointment | ** | skin conditions |

* often used in combination with other materials
** TV less than 1

hints and recommended appropriate patented compounds and products for a variety of human and animal health problems. Their knowledge became a vital source of up-to-date information for isolated regions without easy access to the services of doctors and veterinarians. Often their visit might result in a request for an evening's accommodation for themselves and their horse, but in return children were given candy treats and the homemaker was offered a gift of her choosing from a variety of household products. These gifts were much appreciated by the entire household, and such visits were a special and highly anticipated event.

The most recognizable and frequently encountered group of salesmen were those selling Watkins or Rawleigh products. They offered a wide range of patent medicines, veterinary supplies, fly sprays, spices, and other household products not regularly stocked by the local general store. Medicated ointments and liniments could be used for a variety of health problems, and some could be used on both humans and animals. Many of these medications were complex herbal tinctures, not unlike those prepared in traditional medical practice. Some of these preparations might contain relatively harmless ingredients, but their alcohol content made the person using them feel better. They were identified and used as the "poor person's medicine," and if not entirely harmless, they did provide some relief. The gradual decline in acceptance and use of patent medicines closely paralleled the decline in use of home remedies. Doctors and drugs became not only more available, but also the preferred mode of treatment.

A variety of spices (spetsiia), such as cloves, mustard, and caraway seeds, were also available from such salesmen and from the general store. Both also sold chemicals such as powdered sulphur, blue stone (copper sulphate), alum, and other ingredients that could be used in home remedies.

Of the products (Table 24) purchased from travelling salesmen, druggists, or general merchandisers, ointments and salves were most widely used for relief of external pain and internal congestion. Vaseline was often used as a substitute for animal fats in treating skin conditions. Iodine was used as a skin antiseptic, and camphor oil and Hoffmann's Drops (a patent medicine) treated congestion problems.

## COMMUNITY RESOURCES

Farm newspapers and magazines, both Ukrainian (*Canadian Farmer, Ukrainian Voice, Kanadiysky Rusin* [Canadian Ruthenian], later renamed *Kanadiysky Ukrainetz* [Canadian Ukrainian]) and English *(Winnipeg Free Press)*, printed articles on health issues and home remedies. Subscribers shared simple remedies and treatments for dealing with common health problems. Norah Lewis's paper (see Selected Readings) titled "Goose Grease and Turpentine: Mother Treats the Family's Illnesses" is a nice summary of such helpful tips. The Prosvita Society, a public cultural and educational organization founded in the nineteenth century in Ukraine, published (in Ukrainian) a helpful Canadian medical booklet called *What to Do When the Doctor is not Available.* It discussed

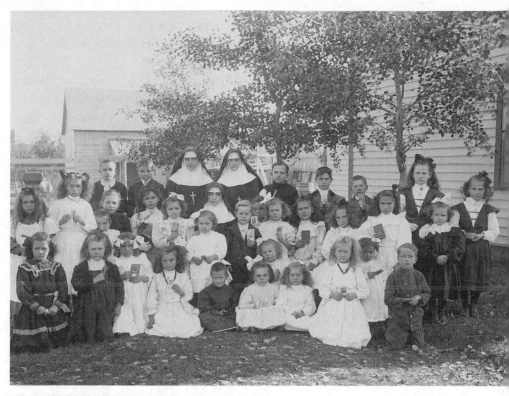

Nuns provided settlers with both spiritual and healing guidance. [PAA B3745]

various health principles and described a range of home remedies for treating common ailments.

> In the early days, the Free Press (Winnipeg newspaper) contained many letters written by its readers on the use of home remedies. Our neighbour had a baby that developed a high fever (vysoka hariachka), and the doctor did not think it would live. The mother remembered one of these "letter remedies" that used a warm onion (tepla tsybulia) plaster. She quickly chopped up and heated some onions, placed these between two pieces of cloth, and put this "plaster" on the baby's chest and back. She applied it regularly for a few days. When the doctor came back to check up on the baby, its fever was down and it was smiling and doing well. — P. S. / Willingdon

Nuns (Sisters) of various religious orders serving in the Ukrainian settlement areas also used a variety of traditional treatments on the sick or shared these treatments with those seeking advice on medical matters. Later on, when schools were more common in settlement areas, teachers became an important source of health-related information based on conventional medicine. Availability, knowledge, and acceptance of these "modern" medical treatments eventually made traditional healing practices seem primitive, embarrassing to use, and less effective in dealing with a family's health problems. Families wanted the best for their children, so conventional medicine won and kitchen medicine lost.

Language was a significant barrier to sharing traditional healing practices with other ethnic groups, as well as with the Aboriginal peoples who annually migrated through settlement areas. Ukrainian settlers living near reserves, however, did have a greater opportunity to learn about local Native peoples' healing agents and remedies—many of which proved to be highly effective. Despite the lack of a common language, both groups saw themselves as being displaced and generously shared their healing skills and other resources.

*The Indians told us a cure for a boil* (chyriak). *You had to go to a black poplar tree, squeeze out some pus from the boil, and rub it on the trunk. As you were doing this you had to say, "So that you can rule here* (tak shchob ty tut panuvav)." *Our neighbours tried this and said that it worked.*
— D. A. / Vegreville

# EIGHT

# Traditional Healing Practices

## GENERAL

Ukrainian home remedies were relatively simple in their preparation and application. They were based on using household and homestead materials that were readily available throughout the year. Most ingredients were common household food items (potato, cabbage, garlic), kitchen materials (salt, flour, honey), or local plant material (wormwood, coltsfoot, yarrow, puffballs) used fresh (summer) or dried (winter). Various home treatments also used body manipulation (massage, bloodletting) or applications of liquids or other materials, primarily to relieve pain.

Liquid remedies (Table 25) generally consisted of soaking in, or steaming with, hot water for external aches and pains (see description in chapter eight). Internal upset or pain was alleviated with various hot tea preparations. Both warm- and cold-water immersion were used for reviving frozen skin. Use of human urine was a common treatment for chapped skin on the feet and hands.

Manipulation-based treatments (Table 26) used a dark warm room to create an effective healing environment for children with chicken pox or measles. A dog's licking was a common treatment for various skin problems. Massage and bloodletting were less common home treatments, because these manipulations were typically provided by specialized folk healers.

Application-based treatments (Table 27) were mainly used in reducing pain or in treating skin conditions. Hot packs and wet or dry cloth wraps were used to reduce aches and pains. Soil or clay was used in treating various skin irritations. Snow or ice was used to thaw frozen skin (a treatment now known to cause

TABLE 25   Treatment Value of liquids used in home healing practices

| Treatment | Treatment Value | Major Application(s) |
|---|---|---|
| Hot water* (soak) | 46 | puncture wounds / rheumatism / cold and flu / infections |
| Hot tea* | 44 | diarrhea / internal pain / sore throat / fever |
| Steam bath* | 31 | rheumatism / chest congestion / cold and flu / muscle aches / chilled body |
| Warm water | 25 | frozen skin |
| Cold water | 23 | frozen skin / burns |
| Facial steaming* | 16 | nasal congestion / breathing problems |
| Human urine | 10 | warts / skin conditions |
| Salt-water (gargle) | 4 | sore throat |
| Horse drool | ** | warts |
| Human saliva | ** | warts / sleeplessness in children |
| Rainwater (off roof) | ** | ringworm |
| Soapy water | ** | head lice |

* sometimes used in combination with other materials
** TV less than 1


more harm than benefit: it may be that the vigorous rubbing associated with the application was what helped the skin to thaw).

Many of the manipulation and application home remedies revealed a low Treatment Value factor, which indicated their use as either not being a traditional practice, of limited use, or possibly acts of desperation in attempting to use or create a treatment that would provide relief. A child treading on an adult's sore back may be one such example. Burning or cutting off warts were extreme and potentially unsafe treatment methods, but did produce faster results than more traditional remedies. Using saliva to treat warts or sleeplessness may simply have been coincidental associations that were considered curative but were not widely used. Applications of a red cloth to treat chicken pox may have been based on healing traditions using a supernatural element or borrowed from other cultures. Similarly, applying fur to a ringworm infection or placing a garter snake on a swollen throat may have been based on Native healing techniques. Some of the traditional Ukrainian home remedies and treatments, such

TABLE 26    Treatment Value of manipulation-based home healing practices

| Treatment | Treatment Value | Major Application(s) |
|---|---|---|
| Warm dark room | 15 | chicken pox / measles |
| Licking by a dog | 10 | ringworm / infections / eye conditions / boils |
| Massage | 7 | muscle aches and pains / abdominal strain / birthing |
| Bloodletting | 5 | "bad" blood / muscle pain / breathing problems |
| Vomiting | 4 | poisoning / hangover |
| Combing of hair | 3 | head lice |
| Cloth probe | 3 | eye debris |
| Tying off | 3 | warts |
| Tongue probe | 3 | eye debris |
| Finger in throat | 3 | inducement of vomiting |
| Cut out/off | 3 | boils / warts |
| Burn | 2 | warts |
| Feather massage | * | infections |
| Rolling on ground | * | muscle pain |
| Bacon on string | * | sore throat |
| Treading on back | * | backache |

* TV less than 1

as bloodletting, cupping, and use of leeches, required specialized materials and more complex treatment preparations. Many of these more specialized treatments required a sequence of applications.

## SPECIALIZED

## *Bloodletting*

A wide range of health problems, such as fatigue, insomnia, inflammation, fever, headaches, chest pains, and epilepsy, were attributed to the accumulation of "bad" blood. This dark, thick blood was thought to congest in specific organs or

TABLE 27    Treatment Value of application-based home healing practices

| Treatment | Treatment Value | Major Application(s) |
|---|---|---|
| Hot pack | 70 | earache / muscle aches / chest congestion / toothache / menstrual cramps / abdominal strain / rheumatism |
| Cloth (wet) wrap* | 61 | headache / fever / sore eyes / cuts / inflamed tonsils / sore throat |
| Cups / pots | 46 | muscle aches and pains / abdominal strain / "bad" blood / chilled body / headache |
| Cloth (dry) wrap | 31 | cuts / sore throat / inflamed tonsils |
| Hot / warm cloth* | 31 | puncture wounds / rheumatism / infections |
| Soil or clay | 22 | cuts / diaper rash / chapped skin |
| Snow / ice | 10 | frozen skin |
| Chimney soot* | 8 | skin conditions / cuts / boils / rheumatism |
| Knife blade | 6 | insect bites |
| Burning cloth | 5 | earache |
| Ashes | 5 | cuts |
| Pipe tar | 5 | ringworm / toothache |
| Tobacco smoke | 4 | earache |
| Human feces | 2 | ringworm |
| Suction | 1 | boils |
| Blanket / quilt wrap | ** | fever |
| Flour | ** | boils |
| Earwax | ** | ringworm |
| Fur | ** | burns |
| Garter snake | ** | swollen throat |
| Linen strap | ** | abdominal strain |
| Red cloth | ** | chicken pox |

* sometimes used in combination with other materials
** TV less than 1

regions of the body and produce severe and prolonged pain in the area. Getting a chill, from wearing inadequate clothing or footwear in cold weather was considered to be a major cause of its formation. Chilling led to isolated and chronic pain in the back, shoulders, chest, and legs. Inflamed varicose veins, and even inflamed nipples during lactation, were also associated with such "bad" blood. Its collection in the head was considered to cause nervousness, tension, and severe headaches. Accumulation of "bad" blood in the limbs produced swollen hands and feet. Elderly women believed that once a woman stopped menstruating (during menopause), "bad" blood accumulated and created many of her chronic ailments.

It was widely accepted that bloodletting (phlebotomy or venesection), which removed such undesirable blood, alleviated the painful conditions it produced. Another method of removing "bad" blood was through the use of cups placed over the skin of these painful areas. A vacuum was created by heating the cups, drawing the blood to the surface, allowing it to be removed from the affected body tissues. If the skin had been cut prior to the placement of the cups, this technique was termed "wet" cupping, and if the skin was not cut it was termed "dry" cupping. Leeches were another method of removing such "bad" blood. These two techniques were widely used by the Ukrainian settlers, with leeches used more often because they were more readily available from local water bodies. Cups were more specialized devices and typically required the service of a folk healer for their proper use. (The various bloodletting techniques are described in chapter eight.)

*If someone suffered from lower back or kidney pain* (holiucha nyrka), *this was said to be due to "bad" blood collecting in the area. This condition was treated with cups, which caused this blood to be drawn to the surface of the skin. This helped the aching to stop. I often saw my mother putting cups* (banky) *on my dad's back in order to relieve such pain* (bil). — L. K. / Star

In the Old Country, bloodletting was a service provided by travelling folk healers and was an accepted medical procedure in the 1800s and early 1900s. In Canada, the technique was most often done by men who had some Old Country familiarity, or even training, in the procedure. These folk healers made regular trips into the Ukrainian settlement areas and provided the service, for a fee, in the patient's home. Each cup was applied at a cost of 25 cents. Later on, a flat fee of $5 to $10 was charged for a full treatment.

Bloodletting *(krovopuskannia)* was generally used by the elderly to deal with a variety of painful old-age ailments, primarily those associated with arthritis and rheumatism. Some individuals used the procedure as a preventative or revitalizing therapy that they had done on a regular six- or twelve-month basis. Many elderly people, through extensive personal experience with the technique, knew how to remove "bad" blood with both cups and leeches. They used ordinary household drinking or shot glasses and locally caught leeches. These items were also available, by mail order, from Eaton's in Winnipeg. The Sisters at the convent in Mundare also provided both of these traditional treatments to people in the surrounding areas.

> *Older people said that applying cups drew out the chilled blood* (zastudena krov). *A woman in our area went around and provided this treatment. Leeches were also used to draw out "blue" blood* (synia krov), *which formed when people got chilled walking barefoot. I remember walking barefoot in some water and leeches attached to my legs. I pulled them off and placed them in a bottle of water for later use. When the leech was placed on the body, it would find the "bad" blood and remove it. People* (liudy) *could also buy leeches, but these had to be ordered from Winnipeg.*
> — M. M. / Vegreville

CUTTING

Bloodletting was typically done using a single-bladed lancet or a two- to three-bladed fleam, which was used to make a small cut *(nadriz)* on one or more large external veins at the top of the foot or the bottom of the wrist. A prescribed amount of blood was then collected in a metal or porcelain bleeding bowl, often marked off to indicate the amount of blood to be collected. The "bad" blood, which appeared dark and thick, was drained into a large white enamel bowl. Blood flow was stopped when "good" or "healthy" blood, which was red and thinner, appeared. The amount of blood removed was typically from one half to one and a half pints, but often the amount was in direct proportion to the donor's overall size and health. Removal of larger amounts of blood, such as a quart or more, was risky, because it would weaken the patient and possibly produce shock. Death was highly unlikely unless the person providing the procedure was inexperienced or if the patient was quite elderly or in extremely poor health.

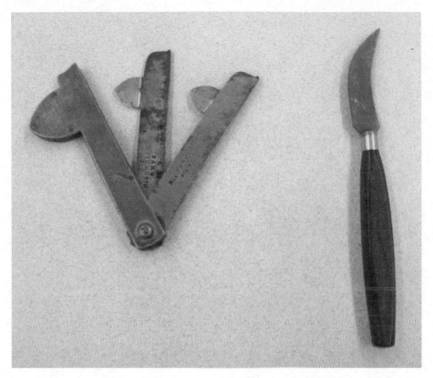

A multi-bladed fleam (left) or a lancet (right) was used for bloodletting. [M. MUCZ]

## CUPPING

For cupping, specialized glass, ceramic, tin, or brass cups were used. The most common were made of thick glass, had a short neck, and were round on the bottom. If such cups were not available, regular drinking glasses or liquor shot glasses could be substituted. The cup's rim was greased to produce a complete seal, and a vacuum was created in the cup to draw the "bad" blood to the skin surface. Heating a cup in a warm oven; burning fine hemp fibres *(volokna vid honopli)* in the cup; rubbing the inside of the cup with alcohol and setting it on fire; burning a candle or match inside the cup; or placing the cup over a lit match stuck in a piece of bread or potato positioned on the skin could be used to rid the cup of air. The suction of the created vacuum drew the "bad" blood to the skin's surface. If the skin had been cut with a multi-bladed scarificator before the cups were put in place, then blood was drawn into the cup and later disposed of. This was "wet" cupping. If no cuts were used ("dry" cupping), this

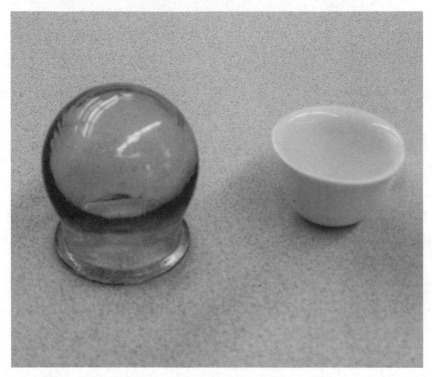

Special small glass (left) or ceramic (right) cups were used to draw out "bad" blood. [M. MUCZ]

caused a large, raised dark welt to develop on the skin covered by the cup. Cups were generally applied to the upper back, chest, and arms. As few as five to eight large cups could be used or as many as forty to eighty small cups, depending on which type was available. In most cases, pain relief was felt immediately after the treatment and would last for a considerable time thereafter. These treatments were applied more than once to achieve a more lasting result.

Dry cupping, which was less invasive and thus safer, was most common. The welts of coagulated blood, equivalent to that of a bad bruise, broke down naturally and in time were absorbed by the body. Another method was to use the dry cup technique first and then to lacerate or prick the welts after the cups were removed. Less commonly, leeches were used to remove the welted blood. The variations probably reflected the personal preferences of the practitioner or the regional (Old Country) preferences of the patient.

*My mother applied cups when an adult had continuous aches and pains*
*common with rheumatism. The cups were either heated or else they had alcohol*
*(alkohol) smeared inside, which was then lit. They were quickly placed on the*
*painful area, but the skin was not cut to let out the bad blood. People always felt*
*better after this treatment.* — C. O. / Edmonton

### LEECHES

Leeches, used for bloodletting, were either the small non-medicinal local varieties caught in local water bodies, or were the larger purchased medicinal types. The latter were regularly stocked by drugstores, but were also available by mail order from suppliers such as Eaton's in Winnipeg. They were typically applied to the lower back, feet, hands, or forehead. Some people even applied them to impacted and swollen gums. As few as two to three, or as many as a dozen, would be applied to the painful or affected area. They would locate the area with the "bad" blood and attach themselves to feed. They were kept in position with a moist towel, and when they were fully gorged (20 to 60 ml of blood), they fell off or were removed manually. If continued bleeding at the incision site was desired, then a hot pack was applied to the area. If bleeding was to be stopped, a pinch of alum was often used. The leeches were then squeezed between the fingers or rolled in salt to make them regurgitate the blood, and then were placed in a jar of slough or pond water for later use. Leeches could remain alive for long periods of time and so were used throughout the year.

*Mother used a leech to draw off blood (krov) from a sore and inflamed gum.*
*She took a hollow spindle, place the leech inside, and put the tube on the sore*
*area. The leech attached and drew off the "bad" blood but was not able to move*
*anywhere else.* — M. K. / Vegreville

## Abdominal Pots

Women, because of numerous pregnancies and demanding daily physical work, often suffered from strained and weakened abdominal muscles, which produced chronic abdominal discomfort and pain. This development was often treated by elderly women who knew how to do abdominal massage and apply pots, using a technique similar to that of cupping, to the affected area.

An earthenware pot, large cup, crock, basin, or even a large tin can could be used. The rim was rubbed with grease to provide a seal, and the inside air was removed by burning hemp fibre residues inside the container. Air could also be removed by placing the container over lit matches embedded in slices of potato that had been placed on the abdomen. The vacuum created in the container caused the abdominal muscles to be raised and tightened. After the containers were removed, unsalted butter, vegetable oil, or a tincture of burdock roots was thoroughly massaged into the area. In less severe cases of abdominal strain, only the massaging treatment might be required. The treated abdominal region was then tightly bandaged with strips of linen cloth and the woman was advised to stay in bed for a half to full day. In severe cases of strain, the treatment was applied over three consecutive days and heavy lifting was not permitted for one and a half to two months. Even doctors were known to recommend this therapeutic treatment when their conventional healing methods proved ineffective.

> There was an older woman (stara zhinka) in our area who knew how to treat someone who strained (natiahnuv) their abdomen and was suffering severe internal pain. She massaged the area and used a large glass jar (sloik) to apply suction to the area. This pulled the strained and collapsed muscles up, which reduced the pain and helped with the healing. — P. K. / Vegreville

## Ear Candling

Good hearing was important to the settlers, and they recognized the ear to be a delicate body structure. Dirty field working conditions and limited opportunities for maintaining proper hygiene meant that keeping the inner ear clean was challenging. Plugged ears could result in bad headaches and lead to temporary hearing loss. It was not uncommon for adults to keep the ear canal clean by regular "candling." The treatment was applied by someone who knew how to do it, generally the mother or grandmother.

The procedure involved taking a small waxed cloth, often the waxy cleaning rag used in decorating Easter eggs, and shaping it into a long, thin funnel. The small opening was inserted into the outer ear canal. The face was protected with a towel or piece of cloth, and the rim of the large open end was lit. The "candle" was allowed to gradually burn down about two thirds of its length and then the flame was extinguished. The burning process created a vacuum in the funnel, which pulled out any debris (wax, dirt, foreign materials) from the inner ear canal and into the funnel itself. The remaining part of the candle, with the accumulated debris, was discarded. Superstitious individuals secretively buried the waste materials so they would not continue to be affected by them.

*My father was in much pain with a bad earache* (bil u vusi), *and we sent for an old man who knew how to treat the problem. He brought a piece of linen cloth and some beeswax* (visk), *which he rubbed onto the cloth. He rolled up the waxed cloth into a funnel shape, about half a foot long, and placed its narrow end into the ear. The area around the ear was covered with towels and then the upper edge of the funnel was lit. As the funnel burned, the old man recited what seemed to be a prayer. The flame* (zapal) *went out when the funnel was half burnt and the remaining part was pulled out of the ear. The funnel was full of some kind of material. The old man carefully rolled up the funnel and its contents. He said he would bury it in a place where people did not walk. Father's pain was gone completely and he fell asleep easily.* — M. B. / Warspite

## Heat Treatments

Traditional Ukrainian folk medicine held the view that getting any body part chilled or cold was the source of chronic and debilitating pain in the affected area. Inducing sweating to counteract such developments was the common treatment for such conditions, based on the idea that a higher body temperature offset the chilling effects of the lower outside temperatures. Higher body temperature does increase blood and lymph fluid circulation, which assists the body in healing itself. Fever is also the body's natural immune-based defensive reaction to bacterial and viral infections. Higher body temperatures are known to greatly restrict the growth of infectious microbes.

The most commonly used heat treatment for chronic aches and pains was to heat up the body and keep it warm for an extended period. This was done by keeping the person in bed, or better yet on the sleeping platform of the indoor clay oven *(pich)*, and covering them with quilts and blankets. A more direct method was to have the affected person sit near a hot stove or oven, fully clothed—possibly in a heavy sheepskin coat. Adults, especially men, would also try to induce additional internal heating by eating bread covered with crushed garlic *(chasnyk)* and pork fat *(solonyna)*. This was commonly washed down with whisky, preferably the stronger medicinal homebrew variety, which also provided internal warming. Children, possessing a more delicate nature and being fussier eaters, were given the crushed garlic in warm milk.

Other heat-based treatments required more extensive preparation. Hot baths and steam baths were used to heat the whole body, while hot compresses, hot packs, and facial steaming were used to warm specific body parts. These heat treatments reduced inflammation or pain and loosened the tension in strained muscles.

### HOT COMPRESSES

Large pieces of soft cloth (flannel was preferred over linen) or coarse towels were soaked in relatively hot water or herbal infusion. These were then wrung out, folded to form a pad, and applied to the affected area. The skin could also be protected by rubbing on vegetable oil or grease prior to applying the wet compress. Moisture helped the heat to penetrate into the body. The hot compress was then covered with a dry cloth or towel to retain the heat, and was then wrapped or bandaged in place. The compress did not retain its heat long and needed to be reheated and reapplied at regular intervals to provide maximum benefit.

### HOT PACKS

These preparations, although similar to the use of a hot water bottle, held their heat much longer and also could be moulded to the affected body part. The heated materials were typically small grains such as **oats** *(oves)*, barley *(iachmin)*, or any coarsely ground cereal *(otruby)*. Salt or fine sand could also be used. These dense materials, except for the ground grain and salt, were placed in a bowl or pan, often soaked in water, and heated in the oven. The heated materials were then placed in a flour or sugar sack or a pillowcase and tied off. The hot pack was then wrapped in a towel to keep it from burning the skin. The patient would either lie on it, have it placed on their chest or back, or have it wrapped around the sore arm or leg. The hot pack was kept on the painful area for one half to one hour for a child, or for an adult as long as four hours or overnight. Such packs were reusable and required only reheating. When an adult needed a longer or more intensive heat treatment, flat rocks, bricks, or a round iron stove plate coverlid would be used.

A hot pack for a baby or a very small child was usually made with eight to ten onion slices heated and softened in boiling water. Boiled flax seeds, when softened and swollen, could also be used. These materials were then placed between moistened folds of woollen or flannel cloth and additionally wrapped in a dry towel. The heated pad was then firmly wrapped onto the chest or back and left on for a short time.

> If anyone in our family (rodnia) had chest congestion, a hot barley bag was used to treat it. Barley was heated in a pan placed in the oven and then the hot barley was placed into a cloth bag. A piece of moist flannel cloth was placed on the chest and the hot bag of barley placed on top. A towel was placed over the bag to keep the heat (teplota) in. The steam and heat helped to loosen up the congestion.
> — A. W. / Daysland

## HOT BATHS

A therapeutic hot bath was used by adults, but this was not common because of the considerable space and preparation it required. A tub (vanna) or a barrel (bochka) was brought into the house and water had to be collected and boiled. This was done in the kitchen, where space and privacy were both limited. A hot bath did provide considerable relief for aching body parts and also provided emotional relaxation. Herbs, such as nettle, chamomile, or flax, or bran were often added to the water for an added therapeutic effect. After a soaking of one half to one hour, the skin was dried with towels and a liniment was applied to provide additional heating. The bather went to bed, was well covered, and stayed warm and relaxed for the rest of the night.

## BODY STEAMING

Steam baths were mostly used by the elderly to obtain some relief from their arthritic and rheumatic pains. These treatments were taken either regularly, as often as three to four times a week for severe pain, or as infrequently as a couple of times a year as a seasonal tonic. A fall steaming, before the first snow came, was used to ward off winter's potential illnesses. A steaming in the spring, after the snow had melted, was used to prepare for an "awakening" or "renewed life" in the season ahead. Used as a tonic, steaming was typically done three times during the same day.

A formal separate steam bath house or shed, common to Scandinavian and Russian settlers, was not used by Ukrainians. Taking a steam bath meant using heated field stones in a large washtub or barrel. The bottom of the container would be covered in a shallow layer of water. In some cases aromatic herbs, such as yarrow, sage, mint, chamomile, nettle, thistle, hemp, birchbark and birch leaves, or hay residue, were added to the water as a healing infusion. The hot rocks, which were often wrapped in wire to make them easier to handle, were then placed in the water to create steam. A stool, webbed chair, or board was placed in or on the container so the bather could sit over the steaming water. A simpler and faster method was to place hot rocks in a bucket of water beside the bather, who was then covered, from their shoulders down, with blankets, sheets or towels. This caused the steam, as it rose, to heat the entire body. An individual could remain in such a steam "tent" for ten to fifteen minutes, depending on their level of heat tolerance. After the steaming treatment, the sore areas of the body could be further stimulated by vigorous beating with young willow or birch twigs. After being dried, the body could be rubbed down with an alcohol and soap mixture, or a liniment (Watkins or Rawleigh) product. The bather then went to bed, was covered with blankets, and stayed warm for the rest of the night.

*My father was very badly crippled by arthritis, and taking a steam bath gave him some relief from the pain. My mother would heat stones (kaminnia) in a pot on the stove and then add water. Father would sit on a chair in which the*

*seat webbing had been removed and the steaming pot of hot water was placed*
*under the seat opening. Father was covered with two large blankets* (kovdra) *and*
*you would soon see sweat running off his face* (lytse). *He would try to do this*
*steaming two to four times a week, depending on how available my mother was to*
*help him set up the materials for the bath.* — J. L. / Mundare

## FACIAL STEAMING

This steam application was a simple, quick, and effective treatment for nasal,
sinus, and chest congestion and could also be used to treat headaches. Boiling
water was placed in a large bowl, and aromatic herbs, such as yarrow or chamomile, or liniment could be added for more effect. The person sat in front of the
bowl, but not over it, and a large towel was placed over their head and the steaming bowl. This allowed the hot, moist air to rise and be slowly inhaled. The face
was never placed directly over the bowl, because the steam would burn the skin.

*People with bad breathing problems* (paskudne dykhannia) *steamed*
*themselves with a basin of hot water into which they put plant materials. These*
*materials were actually barn hay* (sino) *screenings, bits and pieces of herbs and*
*grasses, which were collected and saved for such use. The head* (holova) *was*
*placed near the steaming bowl, covered with a towel, and the rising steam was*
*breathed in.* — J. M. / Camrose

## *Spiritual Healing*

Folk medicine often used spiritual *(dukhovnyi)* and superstitious *(zabobonnyi)*
elements to enhance the healing effectiveness of its treatments. These added
components helped both the healer and the patient to believe and expect that
the folk remedy would produce the desired results. These dual features were
historically associated with ancient beliefs that many, if not all, health problems were attributable to evil spirits or to some spiritual transgression. In traditional folk medicine, the roots of most psychological and emotional problems
(nervousness, fitful sleep, anxiety, unprovoked crying) are associated with some

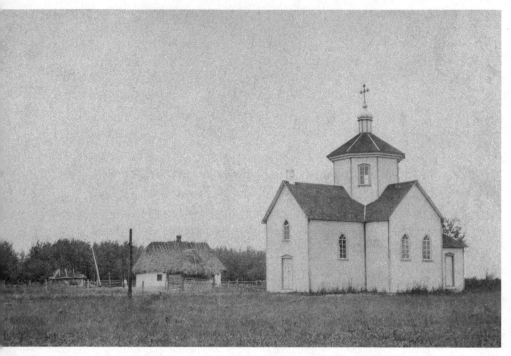

Religion was an important element in Ukrainian bloc settlements. [PAM N11645]

spiritual crisis. Even physical problems, such as warts, were treated with superstitious cures. For Ukrainians, deeply rooted in Christian religious traditions, it
was not uncommon to seek God's healing intervention, or the intercession of
saints and angels, when all other treatments had failed. As folk practices became
more refined and materially based, these spiritual elements assumed a lesser
role. Resident spiritual healers were acknowledged for their abilities and were
frequently sought out in dealing with problems for which material-based folk
remedies were ineffective.

Superstitious practices, based on pre-Christian as well as Christian beliefs,
were also applied to the gathering, preparation, and application of certain healing materials. The time of day, phase of the moon, or a holy day, were considered
to influence the healing effectiveness of the gathered materials. Bitter-tasting
herbs, such as wormwood, were considered to be more effective in counteracting
negative spiritual influences on poor health. Objects such as water, candles, and

incense, blessed by a priest, were believed to be holy and to therefore possess additional healing powers.

In some folk treatments, prayers or other religious incantations were recited during the procedure. Prescribed healing agents would typically be taken three times a day, or treatments applied over three consecutive days, to invoke the Holy Trinity in the healing process. Treatments might also have healing ingredients used in multiples of three or in some combination of twelve, which represented the number of Christ's apostles. Such belief systems and practices, especially strong in the elderly, reflected Old Country traditions and religious practices. It must also be remembered that the majority of the folk healers were elderly women, and they did things the way they had been taught in the Old Country.

Objects such as water, flowers, foliage, and knives were also regularly blessed during various religious holy days. These blessed, and now holy, items often served as the last treatment resource when all else had failed. They were most commonly used for the very young or the very old to inspire additional hope for a miraculous cure. Although they could be administered by any family member, they were most often applied by an elderly person with a deep and strong faith. Such individuals were considered to be "blessed" *(blahoslovennyi)* by God with a divine healing ability.

The preventative or healing powers of these blessed objects were always invoked with a prayer, which was characteristically repeated three times and sought God's intercession on the sick person's behalf. Blessed natural materials, such as flowers, that had been used in healing were never simply discarded— they were always respectfully disposed of by being burned or buried.

## HOLY WATER

Holy water was blessed on the Feast of Jordan *(Iordan),* held on Epiphany (January 19). It was distributed to each family attending that service and was taken home in a small scaler or jar. Each family member immediately consumed a portion to maintain good health in the coming year. This would help ward off evil and restore health in the event of a serious illness. The remaining holy water was kept for future healing or blessing purposes. When used for healing, the sick person was typically given a small amount of holy water to drink, or it was sprinkled and rubbed onto their face or body. Eye conditions, which were serious health problems with limited folk remedies, were often treated by washing the affected eye with holy water. Warts were also treated with holy water, but it had to be applied on a day with a full moon. Warts could also be treated with water thrown over a straw roof on St. John's Day *(na Ivana)* (July 7). This water was allowed to drip onto the wart in order to remove it. In desperation, holy water was widely used in the Ukrainian community as both a preventative and curative agent during the influenza pandemic of 1918-1919.

> *There was an older man* (starshyi cholovik) *living near us who healed people with prayer* (molytva). *People came to him when all other treatments were not helping. He washed their face with holy or blessed water and then prayed over them. He would only do this healing when the moon* (misiats) *was old—that is, full.* — E. L. / Two Hills

## BLESSED PLANTS

Blessed plants *(sviata roslyna)* were dried and kept available for use throughout the year. Flowers were blessed at the Feast of Transfiguration in the fall; pussy willows (catkins) were blessed at Easter time in the spring; and a variety of foliage was blessed during Green holy days *(zeleni sviata)*—Pentecost Sunday and St. John's Day in the summer. Blessed pussy willow and blessed Easter bread *(paska)* could be used as a poultice on unhealthy eyes. Willow catkins could also be swallowed as a preventative measure for throat problems. Other dried blessed foliage could be soaked and used in a poultice for boils or on poorly healing infected sores. Some blessed plants were used to make a tea for difficult-to-treat stomach problems. Blessed flowers could also be soaked in water and the liquid used internally or externally on a person with a serious or prolonged illness such as cancer. Blessed plant materials could also be burned, and the healing smoke wafted over the sick person's head, as a final desperate healing measure.

## BLESSED KNIFE

A blessed knife *(blazhennyi nizh)*, consecrated along with food during the Easter service, was also used as a healing instrument. It could be rubbed on persistent skin lumps, applied to aching teeth, or touched to three sides of a seriously ill person's body. Blessed knives, other similarly blessed household utensils (spoons or ladles), or smoke from the burning of blessed vegetation were used to protect the family and homestead against severe hail and thunderstorms.

## Sympathetic Healing

A treatment that appears to have no medical or pharmacological healing basis is termed a "sympathetic" treatment or cure. It relies on the concept of a placebo effect, in which the harmless and therapeutically ineffective material or treatment somehow contributes to the sick person's recovery. This practice is based on the patient's forming a strong belief, because of what is given or being done, that the intervention will contribute to their recovery. The importance of the patient's psychological role in the healing process is not well understood but is, however, recognized to be important. Any treatment, in whatever form, is seen as a positive action from the ill person's perspective and helps them to believe that they will get better. The Roman philosopher Seneca observed that part of any cure is the patient's "wish or desire" to be cured. Such a healing feature is especially important in children, who possess not only a natural fear of being sick, but also a relatively low pain threshold. In addition to whatever effectiveness a natural treatment might provide, a mother's caring touch and expressed concerns, coupled with prayers said on the child's behalf, would have a strong impact on the child's belief that he or she should and would get better.

Sympathetic healing would have been important to the pioneers, because the basis, whether viral (colds) or physiological (aches), of most health problems was unknown and typically associated with superstitious causes (aches due to chilling or "bad" blood). Many of these conditions would, in time, heal without intervention because of the body's natural healing capabilities. Drinking sufficient amounts of fluids, eating nutritious foods, and having adequate rest are major factors in enabling the body to "heal itself." Most common everyday health problems, such as colds, headaches, and digestive upset, run their course, and full recovery typically occurs in a matter of days without additional treatment. Folk healing relies extensively on the use of various biological and non-biological materials whose specific roles in the healing process remain unclear but which nevertheless are highly effective in overcoming the health problem being treated. The curative powers of these various healing materials and treatments undoubtedly extend beyond the actual curative properties of their ingredients because of the associated sympathetic healing factor their use creates.

> *A young child* (moloda dytyna) *had an infected sore on its foot and it was not healing. An older woman treated it by taking some stiff feathers* (pir'ia) *and stroking them downward on the wound. This caused pus and blood to flow from the infection. After a number of such treatments, the wound began to heal. The child's mother thought that this "massaging" caused the wound to "relax" and start healing on its own.* — J. S. / Lamont

# NINE

# Traditional Healing Preparations

Plants, used medicinally by Ukrainian settlers, were applied whole, mashed up for poultices, or had their active ingredients extracted through liquid preparation. Herbal extracts were used as restorative, preventative, stimulatory, relaxant, or tonic agents. The majority were safe to use, but some (wormwood) are now known to have adverse effects with long-term use, and even in the old days it was advised that they not be used by pregnant or lactating women.

Plant parts were most effective when collected when their active ingredients were considered to be at peak concentrations. Roots and rhizomes were harvested in the fall, bark and twigs in the late winter or early spring, stems and leaves before the flowers formed, flowers when they first opened, and fruits and seeds when ripe. Herbs collected on holy days, such as yarrow, which was to be collected on St. John's Day (July 7), were considered to possess greater healing potential. Only healthy and intact plant parts were collected. They were washed and rinsed, and whenever possible were used in their fresh state. Essential healing plants, such as cranberries, were also dried for use throughout the year. Plant drying was either done slowly in the open shade or rapidly by placing the plants in a clay oven. The dried matter was then hung along the inside eaves, kept in paper bags, or placed in paper-covered jars. Mouldy herbal material was discarded, because it was known to be less effective and possibly dangerous to use.

Most of the traditional healing preparations used by Ukrainian settlers were made from a single plant species and rarely in combination with other species. Extraction of active ingredients depended on the type of herb used, the parts used, the solubility of the healing ingredients in hot or cold water or alcohol,

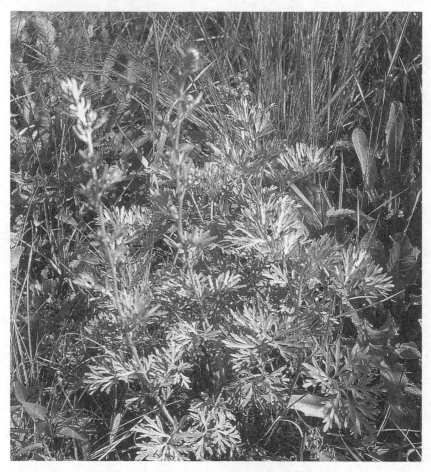

Wormwood tea was bitter but helpful for digestive problems. [M. MUCZ]

the required extract concentration, and the condition being treated. In winter, dry plant parts, primarily roots and berries, were used. In summer, fresh flowers and leaves were considered most effective. Softer plant structures, such as leaves, had their tissue ingredients more easily extracted than did the woodier bark and roots. Water-based extractions were easy to prepare, but had to be used relatively quickly because they spoiled easily. They often kept for only a few days and were stored in a cool, dark place. Alcohol-based extracts were better preserved and could be stored, in a dark bottle, for up to two years.

*My father suffered from a severe heart* (sertse) *condition, high blood pressure, and diabetes* (solodka krov). *Nothing the doctors did for him helped, so in frustration with modern medicine he decided to treat himself. He collected wormwood and boiled it to make a strong extract. The liquid was so bitter* (hirka) *that he could only take one or two teaspoons a day. It seemed to improve the quality of his life greatly and showed the value of home remedies.* — H. M. / Warspite

## INFUSIONS

These liquid preparations, also known as a tea or tisane, could be taken in a variety of ways: directly, heated and their steam inhaled, as a soaking solution, applied indirectly with a wet compress, or massaged into the skin. Most preparations required using hot—but not boiling—water, but cold water was also used. Herbal material—a half to one teaspoon of crushed dry matter or one to two tea spoons of fresh whole plant tissue—was placed in a ceramic or glass cup, and the water was poured over it. The container was covered, to prevent the loss of essential and aromatic oils, and allowed to steep for five to fifteen minutes. Extraction time was proportional to the desired concentration of the extract. Steeping for ten minutes was most common, but tough leaves might require fifteen to thirty minutes. The infusion was then strained through cheesecloth and cooled to a drinkable temperature. Unprocessed **honey** *(med)* or sugar was added if it was to be taken by a child. Adults often drank it with a bit of alcohol, primarily moonshine, for an added medicinal effect. Such infusions could be kept, in a dark and cool place, for a day or two, but were reheated before use.

If heating destroyed or inactivated any of the herb's essential ingredients, cold water or sun extraction was used. This involved placing the plant material in cold water and soaking it overnight, or placing the solution in the sun for a day or two. The infusion was then used in the same way as a hot extraction. These methods, as well as hot or cold oil infusions, were not widely used.

If larger amounts of an infusion were required, as in a healing bath, then seven (dry) to fourteen (fresh) heaping tablespoons of plant material were placed in a pot of boiling water and steeped for an hour. The solution was then strained and added to the bath water. Herbal material could also be placed in a cloth sachet and directly immersed in the bath water for gradual, continual release.

Infusions for fevers and colds were typically taken as hot drinks. Cold ones were used to enhance appetite, increase urine production, or to settle the digestive system. Berry teas were highly effective healing agents, easily made by adding one to two tablespoons of a fruit concentrate to a cup of hot or cold water.

*My brother was born at home, and the midwife who helped deliver him brought some dried chamomile* (romanets). *She had me make some tea with it and asked me to strain it through a cloth. She gave my brother a half a cup of this tea, drop by drop, before he was allowed to nurse on any milk. She said it would clean out his stomach and make him healthy* (zdorovyi). *He was healthy all his life* (zhyttia). — M. S. / Vegreville

## DECOCTIONS

These preparations were extracted, using larger amounts of water and longer boiling periods, from tougher plant parts such as roots, stems, and bark. To a pot (two cups) of **cold** *(zymna)* or boiling water was added two (dry) to four (fresh) teaspoons of finely chopped or ground herbal material. The mixture, left uncovered, was boiled for ten minutes and then simmered for ten more. Sometimes it was not boiled but only simmered for twenty minutes. If a more concentrated solution was needed, the preparation could be simmered for thirty to forty minutes. This reduced the decoction's liquid content by one third to one half, which produced a more concentrated solution. The solution was then strained through a cloth and cooled. It could also be stored, in a covered container, for a few days. Extremely hard plant material, such as bark or pulpy (hawthorn) berries, was placed in boiling water and left in a warm place to extract for as long as twenty-four hours.

Preparing barley or flax-seed water required boiling about two ounces (a handful) of whole or crushed seed in six cups of water. The solution was heated until the volume was reduced by one third to one half, then the thickened decoction was strained. **Honey** or lemon juice *(sik vid tsytryny)* could be added to make the decoction taste better. It was used in small doses, a cupful for an adult or one teaspoon to one tablespoon for a child.

*Mother went and collected chokecherry* (cheremkhy) *branches with the berries* (iahody) *still attached. She dried these and later, when she needed to use them, boiled the berries to soften them up. The soft outer berry layer was scraped off and the rinsed pits were boiled again for another two hours. She strained off this liquid, added sugar* (tsukor), *and then bottled it as a cold and cough remedy* (liky). — M. D. / Vegreville

## TINCTURES

Not all the active ingredients in plant material are water-soluble. Some of the non-mineral and vitamin compounds can be extracted only by being dissolved in a strong (at least 25 to 50 per cent) alcohol such as brandy, vodka, gin, or whisky/**moonshine**. For non-drinkers, vinegar could be used as the solvent, or the alcohol could be diluted (one to three parts) with water. The chopped, cut, or ground plant material was then placed in a clear glass bottle, completely covered with the liquid at a ratio of two parts liquid to one part plant material, and then capped. It was placed in a warm, sunny location inside the house to get the added benefit of the sun's energy, or kept in a dark, cool location for a slower extraction. It was shaken regularly (typically daily) over a two- to six-week period. The solution was then strained and the tincture placed in a dark, stoppered bottle. Because of alcohol's preservative nature, it could be stored and remain effective for as long as two to five years. The tincture, because of its concentrated nature, was not diluted with water and was used only in small portions. It was taken, a teaspoon or tablespoon at a time, directly or added to warm water or tea. It was also not recommended, because of its alcohol content, for pregnant or lactating women, nor was it generally given to children. It could also be used as a liniment rubbed on the skin for easy absorption.

## FRUITS AND JUICES

Fresh or dried, fruits were boiled in water to produce a juice used as a healing remedy. Fruit was also cooked, with sugar or honey added, for a longer period to produce a syrupy concentrate used for healing purposes. Sometimes fruit was simply placed in a jar, covered with sugar or honey, allowed to sit in a warm room for a month or so, and regularly mixed to maximize liquid formation. This healing solution was then strained through a cloth and taken in small portions, one to two tablespoons at a time, three times a day. Fruit concentrates could also be added to a cup of hot or cold water for a tonic-like health drink.

> The lowbush cranberry (kalyna) is better and tastier than the highbush cranberry. Mother always gathered it, cooked it, and put it into crocks. It stored well and was good medicine (medytsyna). I was once very sick with a fever, had a bad stomachache, and could not eat anything. My mother gave me some of the cooked cranberry fruit and I ate it with some bread (khlib). It quickly cured my condition. — P. K. / Vegreville

## POPPY EXTRACT

Homestead work often required both the husband and wife to work together in the fields. Sometimes the wife might need to do chores in the garden or farmyard, and at those times infants and toddlers became significant impediments to getting any work done. Even if they were brought to the work site, they would have to be left unattended but continued to be a source of worry for the mother. At home a fussy infant or sick child might not sleep well, which interrupted sleep for others in the family. Taking an infant or a fussy child to a social event such as a three-day wedding would undermine the parents' ability to enjoy themselves. One parent, typically the mother, would need to devote their time and attention to the child.

In such circumstances, an Old Country practice of "doping" children with a narcotic-based sedative was used. An extract of opium poppy or, less commonly, hemp, was used. Early on, both plants were grown for culinary (oil) purposes and therefore they were always available. Most people were aware of the dangers of using such a strong narcotic, but desperation made its use more common than not. Its frequent and continued use was also known to produce a negative effect on a child's physical and mental development. In cases of extreme use, an affected child could develop learning difficulties and struggle in school. Many informants knew, or had heard of, such mentally handicapped children in their area. These occurrences were associated with desperate, poor, and uneducated families with limited options. Later on (in the 1930s), this practice became rare, because it became illegal to grow opium poppies and hemp. Larger families also meant that older children were available to look after their siblings.

> *I knew a woman who would often use poppy* (mak) *water to get her child to sleep* (spaty) *soundly. She bathed her one-year-old daughter in a solution made by boiling green* (zeleni) *poppy pods in water. It was quite harmful to the child, and she never did learn to talk. Poppies could even kill* (zabyty). *My mother had some poppies growing by the granary, and when a steer ate some of them, it died.*
> — A. C. / Smoky Lake

The poppy sedative *(molochko / makivka)* was an opium poppy infusion. It was made by boiling chopped green (unripe) poppy heads, or ground immature seeds, in water. A quarter cup of poppy material to a cup of water was the proportion most often used. Unripe poppy heads could also be dried for use at other times of the year. Poppy leaves, and less commonly hemp leaves, could also be boiled, but produced a weaker solution. The concentrated liquid extract was kept in a jar and used as required. Depending on a child's size, a few drops, or a few tablespoons, would be given directly or added to the child's water or milk. In about half an hour the child would fall into a deep sleep and, depending on how strong the dose was, easily sleep a full day or more. A child in such a deep sleep could be safely left unattended in the house while both parents worked outside. Unfortunately, the child's long-term well-being was often not considered and was sometimes compromised.

Parents concerned about directly exposing their child to such a deep prolonged sleep used a similar but more controlled form of sedation. Chopped unripe poppy heads, or immature seeds, were mixed with a bit of sugar and tied off in a piece of moist cloth. This makeshift soother provided a milder form of sedation that the child could suck on while awake. A child with such a soother could be left unattended in the house or field. These soothers were also used when infants were taken to social events.

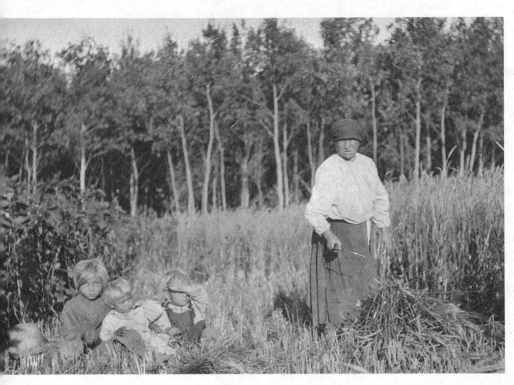
Women working in the field still had to look after their children. [PAM N9697]

*I was a fussy baby* (nemovlia) *and cried a lot. A woman told my mother that there was something that would make me sleep. She told my mother to mash up unripened poppy seeds and place these in a cloth bag, which was then tied up. I was given this moist bag to suck on. The poppy juice did make me sleep well, but it also dulled my mind. When I went to school* (shkola), *my brothers and sisters were doing well, but I was not. Another woman told my mother that it was the poppies that made me a slow learner. My mother cried* (plakala) *when she realized what she had done to me. All she could say was that there was so much work* (robota) *to do and she just needed to keep her baby from crying.* — E. C. / Vegreville

A fussy baby who slept poorly or fitfully could also be given a sedative bath to calm it down. Unripe poppy heads, immature seeds, and/or green leaves were

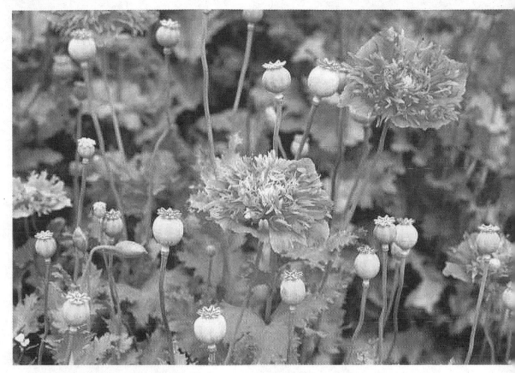

Poppies were grown for seed oil but also could be used to make a sedative tea.
[PHOTO COURTESY OLD DOMINION UNIVERSITY]

boiled in water and the child bathed in the solution. The body absorbed enough narcotic sedative from the bath water to make the child calmer and more manageable. Another alternative was to crush unripe poppy heads or seeds, place these in a moist cloth, and wrap it around the child's forehead or throat. This produced a similar absorptive sedating effect. Less commonly, milky sap (raw opium) was extracted from the green poppy heads or seeds, and a bit was smeared on the child's forehead. It produced a similar sedating effect. A more cautious and concerned mother might simply place unripe poppy seeds directly in a child's pillow or in a piece of cloth that was then placed on the pillow. Use of such milder sedating treatments was atypical because, although less harmful, they were less effective.

Eating unripe poppy seeds, or consuming a few tablespoons of a poppy extract, was also a quick-acting, effective sedative for both sick children and adults. It produced a deep stupor that deadened pain and permitted uninter-rupted rest or sleep. Local elderly healers, familiar with the Old Country rem-edies, prepared such a painkiller by collecting beads of raw opium resin from lacerated poppy heads and dissolving these in alcohol. Such a tincture was used sparingly and only for conditions with excessive and prolonged pain. This prac-tice was not common, because it was recognized that it was highly addictive.

Occasionally, older children ate unripe poppy seeds to experience a tempor-ary state of euphoria. The side effect of such activity, however, was a severely upset stomach and undoubtedly a severe reprimand from parents, who knew of the potential dangers of using such a "drug." Such non-medicinal use of opium poppies, or hemp, was generally uncommon in Ukrainian settlements, but it was not unheard of to have people from the town or city raiding country gardens for such potentially hallucinogenic materials.

## ALCOHOL

Whisky was the form of alcohol most often used in Ukrainian home remedies—usually homebrew, or moonshine, which had been distilled a second time to create a more potent, medicinal-quality product. Homebrew, although illegal, was widely available and brewed throughout all Ukrainian settlement areas. It was mainly used for social functions, but because of its availability in most homes, it was also an important home remedy ingredient. Store-bought alcohol, generally brandy, did not have the potency and taste of well-made homebrew and was also expensive.

During Prohibition (1916–1923), it was illegal to make or possess homebrew. It was, however, lawful to purchase, and have in the household, a quart of hard liquor and a gallon of beer. Steep fines did little to prevent the production and use of homebrew. Legal liquor was available from drugstores, but required a prescrip-tion and was to be used only for medicinal applications. Its purchase involved an initial fee to the doctor for the prescription, and a further payment to the druggist. This made homebrew the preferred alcohol, not only for its taste but also its price. However, during the Prohibition era a large number of prescriptions were written and much alcohol was purchased for supposedly medicinal purposes.

The moonshine considered most effective for home remedies was that which had been distilled twice. The first distillation produced a product with

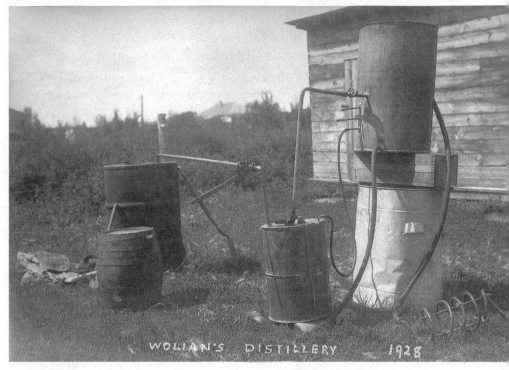

WOLIAN'S DISTILLERY 1928

Homebrew was illegal to make but an important ingredient in home remedies. [PAA G204]

an alcohol content of about 60 per cent, but an additional distillation increased its strength to about 90 per cent. Its potency was tested by burning a sample in a teaspoon. The higher the alcohol content, the longer and more completely the sample burned.

Alcohol, whether purchased or homemade, was used in a variety of home treatments that required warming the body or sedating it. Many elderly men, practising Old Country traditions, drank a shot glass portion (*portsua*) of alcohol daily. When used as a tonic or appetite enhancer, it was also taken in shot-glass portions. Medicinally it was dispensed in shot glass (adult) or teaspoon to tablespoon (child). Alcohol was also used to make tinctures, primarily from wormwood, which was commonly taken for abdominal pain or digestive upset. Pure alcohol was often rubbed into the skin to heat and loosen up sore and aching muscles.

*Dad made moonshine by fermenting a mash of wheat, potatoes, sugar, and*
*yeast for about a week and a half. He distilled this once and then again a second*
*time to make it a stronger (98 proof) alcohol. Mother took a quart of the second*
*distillation for medicinal use. She would rub it on her rheumatic wrists and on*
*any strains or sprains we might get. Dad used the rest of the moonshine for*
*social* (suspilnyi) *purposes.* — M. D. / Vegreville

## POULTICES

These are moistened and crushed masses of **plant** *(roslyna)* or non-plant material
applied directly to the affected area of the skin and wrapped or tied on. They
were used for treating inflammations, fractures, ulcers, boils, skin infections,
wounds, and painful or swollen joints.

In summer, fresh, washed leaf material was used, but in winter dried plant
material was softened in boiling water and then crushed, bruised, or mashed to
release its active ingredients. Plant material could also be made into a paste-like
preparation by adding flour, honey, or cream. This moist, and preferably warm,
mixture was then placed either directly on the skin or between the folds of moistened gauze, linen, or cotton cloth and held in place with strips of cloth. To reduce
irritation, and to make changing the poultice easier, the skin surface could be first
covered with animal fat, unsalted butter, or cream. The most widely used herbal
poultice materials were coltsfoot *(pidlibuk / babka)* and plantain (*podorozhnyk / babka*)
leaves. Non-herbal materials, including clay, grease, and bread, were also used, but
were considered less effective because they contained fewer natural healing agents.

Poultices were often put on at bedtime and kept on overnight. When used
during the day, they were kept fresh by being changed one to three times daily and
were generally used for three to five consecutive days to ensure maximum healing.

*Working on a church roof* (na tserkovnomu dakhu), *I fell off and landed on a*
*four-inch steel spike, which went right through my foot. My friend* (pryiatel), *using*
*pliers, pulled it out. I wrapped the wound and kept on working. A doctor happened*
*to drop by and on hearing of my injury suggested that I go to the hospital where*
*the wound could be cleaned out and treated with medicine. He also suggested that*

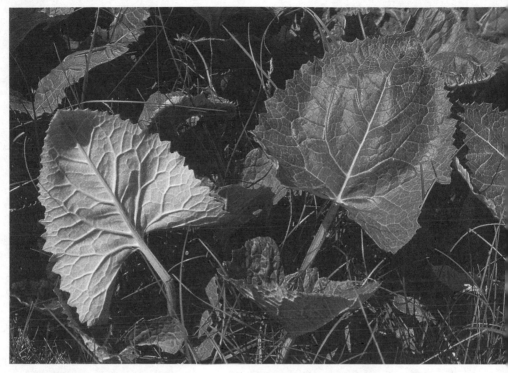

Coltsfoot poultices quickly healed serious flesh injuries. [M. MUCZ]

*I should rest* (vidpochyvaty) *it until it had healed. My friend told me he knew a better and faster home remedy that would have me well in only four days. He told me to get a fresh quart of milk* (moloko) *and some coltsfoot* (pidlibuk) *leaves. These leaves are large, cabbage-shaped, and dark green on top but fuzzy and white below. They were to be soaked whole in the milk for about half an hour. A soaked leaf was to be placed, fuzzy side down, on each side of the wound and wrapped on with a loosely woven cloth so that air could reach the wound. I did this and lay down in a tent to rest. I began to feel the pain* (bil) *in the foot decreasing and I quickly fell asleep. The next morning I awoke, pulled on my boots, and went off to work on the church again. I had completely forgotten about my injury and when reminded of it, I could only see a white* (bilyi) *mark on either side of the foot. The doctor came by later that day and was amazed as to how quickly and well the wound was healing. He now saw for himself how effective traditional remedies were.* — M. K. / Smoky Lake

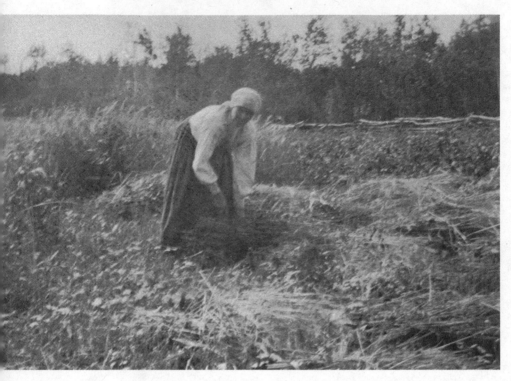

Strenuous physical field work resulted in many aches and pains. [PAM N11662]

## PLASTERS

Plasters were applied to the outer skin, like poultices, but were much larger, put on for a shorter time, and generated considerable heat. They were commonly used in treating colds, chest congestion, and pneumonia-like conditions. Their effect-iveness was in heating up the chest and/or back. This increased blood circulation in the area and quickly broke up accumulated phlegm in the lungs. Their active ingredient was **mustard** *(hirchytsia)*, garlic, or horseradish. Although plasters could be used on young children and even infants, they were mostly used on older children and adults because of the danger of burning the skin if applied too long.

The most commonly used type of plaster was prepared by mixing dry mus-tard with flour in the following proportions: 1:6 (infant), 1:4 (child), and 1:1 to 1:2 (adult). Enough warm water was added to make a thick paste, which was easier to apply and keep on. The paste was spread between a piece of folded brown paper, flannel, or linen cloth. If used on an infant or young child, the delicate skin was first covered with a protective layer of grease, such as **goose fat** *(salo vid husky),* unsalted butter, or Vaseline. The skin was then covered with a piece of moist or dry cloth for added protection. The plaster was placed on top of this protective cloth; covered with an additional cloth; and then wrapped on with strips of cloth, a kerchief, or a towel.

Plaster mixtures with a high mustard content were to be kept on for only ten to fifteen minutes at a time, but weaker ones could be left on for up to thirty or sixty minutes. Men, if extremely congested, might keep an extremely mild plaster on overnight. In any case, the skin was periodically checked to ensure that it was not getting overly red and showing evidence of second-degree burns. After the plaster was removed, the sweaty skin was wiped dry; **goose fat**, liniment, ointment, or camphorated oil was rubbed on; and the patient was kept well-covered with quilts and blankets. The additional bed coverings produced further beneficial heating and sweating. A new plaster was typically reapplied every two or three hours, and for serious congestion, or severe aches, the treatment was used over a two- to three-day period.

*My side (blk) was very painful (bolluchyi), but with all the farm work, it never cleared itself up. I saw a doctor, but whatever he tried did not help. A woman told me to use a mustard and flour* (hirchytsia i muka) *plaster on the area but not to make the mixture too strong. I mixed the two dry materials with warm water, but I added more mustard than flour to the mixture. I put the mixture between a folded cloth and then applied it to the sore area. I quickly felt the skin warming and it soon started to feel hot* (hariacha). *It burned, but I left it on until the evening. When I finally took off the mustard plaster, my skin had burned and was sticking to the cloth. In time the skin did heal, and the pain never returned to the area.* — M. C. / Smoky Lake

A less commonly used, but milder, plaster was prepared with grated horseradish or garlic. The plaster was applied in the same way as a mustard plaster, and for highly tolerant adults was placed directly on the skin. Since the heat generated was not as intense, this type of plaster could be left on for one to three hours, and in some cases overnight. The main disadvantage of these plasters was that when they were removed, they left a strong odour on the skin.

## SALVES

These are semi-solid, non-water soluble, botanically or non-botanically based preparations that are easily absorbed by the skin. Such medicated ointments were a common home remedy of the Bukovinians, who used more woody plant materials in their healing remedies. Salve composition was relatively simple, often nothing more than a healing ingredient (sulphur) suspended in a base material (goose fat). More complex mixtures, using a variety of materials, required greater preparation time. Salve recipes (composition and preparation) were often closely guarded family secrets, but the products were generously shared with anyone who might need them.

More complex salves, with three to five ingredients, also had active healing components that were infused into a base compound such as butter, fat, oil, or Vaseline. Beeswax was often added to the mixture for greater consistency. Proportions of herbal material, fat/oil, and wax were generally disproportionate (4:4 – 6:1), but other mixtures used all ingredients in equal amounts. Proportions varied from family to family. Blessed materials, such as church candle wax drippings and incense, were important additives because they were believed to provide additional supernatural healing powers. Incense, or a conifer (spruce or pine) resin, was added to make the preparation smell more like a medicinal product. This provided an additional psychological (sympathetic) healing element to the salve.

All ingredients were mixed in an enamel pot or bowl, placed over a low heat, and stirred continuously to keep the ingredients well mixed. After an adequate extraction time, which varied from family to family, the mixture was cooled and then strained through a folded piece of cheesecloth. Some healers simply poured the mixture into cold water and collected the salve as it separated out. The solidified material was collected, or scraped, into small ceramic jars or glass bottles and kept covered for later use. Salves had to be stored properly, under cool and dark conditions, or else they would eventually go bad because of their fat or oil content. The salve, a highly effective material, was easily absorbed by the skin and created a protective and soothing cover over the injury.

Salve *(tsiliushcha maz)* formulations varied mainly in the types and amounts of ingredients used. Some typical combinations include:

- beeswax + conifer resin + beef tallow + unsalted butter + incense.
- sweet cream + unsalted butter + beeswax + conifer resin + incense.
- conifer or black poplar resin + vegetable oil + sulphur + sheep fat and brains.
- conifer resin + pig's gallbladder + fat + beeswax.
- conifer resin + sulphur + goose or pork fat.
- unsalted butter + beeswax + conifer resin.
- conifer resin + beeswax + honey + used axle grease.
- conifer resin + beeswax + goose fat or lard.

## OILS

Homemade medicinal oils were basically infusions, using oil instead of water as the extracting agent, of herbal materials or other common household products. A vegetable oil was commonly used, because it required no specific preparation and was always available. Three specialized types of oil-based products (listed below) were also associated with traditional Ukrainian healing practices, but these required special preparation, which meant that they were not always available in a household. It was not uncommon for some local family to have such an oil and to make it available to anyone who needed it.

Specialized oil-based preparations included:

- Cream oil: Fresh sweet cream was gently heated and stirred in a pan until an oil-like residue began to form on its surface. This material, resembling melted butter, was then carefully scooped off with a teaspoon and saved for use on skin conditions that were slow and poor in healing.
- Egg yolk oil: Eggs were boiled until their yolks were quite firm, dark, and showing an oily coating. The oily yolks were removed and crushed to separate out their fine oil residue, which was carefully collected with a teaspoon and stored in a small jar or bottle.

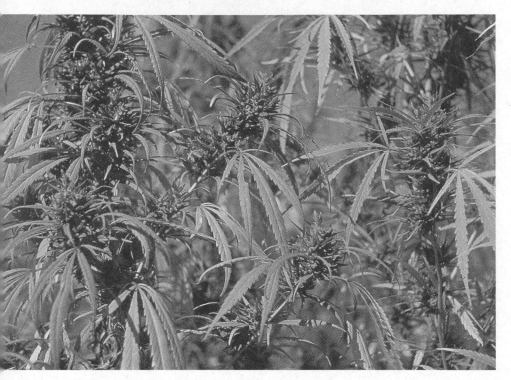
Hemp was used for seed oil and its tough weaving fibre
[PHOTO COURTESY WARD'S NATURAL SCIENCE]

- Hemp seed oil: Regular greenish yellow hemp-seed cooking oil was
  prepared, in a community press, by crushing and pressing hemp
  seeds. It was generally used for treating simple skin problems. More
  serious and difficult-to-heal skin conditions, such as eczema and
  severe rashes, required a special hemp seed oil that required more
  elaborate preparation. This oil was heat extracted from whole seeds
  and required the use of two different-sized unglazed pots or tins.
  One small container, with a lid and perforated base, was fit into a
  larger container. The small pot was loaded one third to one half with
  raw hemp seeds, covered, and wedged into the top of larger pot. The
  assembled pots were then buried just below the soil surface. A fire was
  built over these pots and kept slowly burning for the duration of the
  day. Once the fire died out and the ground had cooled, the pots were

dug up. The large "collection" pot contained the heat-extracted hemp oil. This dark oil was a strong but effective healing agent. It was not to be used on delicate facial skin because it produced an immediate burning sensation and was strong enough to cause skin disfiguration. It was easily stored for later use.

*At home* (vdoma) *we treated skin problems with "soil oil", which my mother had learned how to make in the Old Country. The very dark, blackish oil was extracted by heating hemp seed in the ground with a slow fire. It was kept in a jar and covered with wax paper* (voshchenyi papir). *It was used to treat eczema and other serious skin conditions. When used, it was applied with a wing feather and never with a cloth or finger. When put on it would cause a burning* (hariachyi) *sensation but it did clear the skin problem up.* — P. L. / Willingdon

## FATS

The use of an animal fat, often called grease, in home remedies was also wide-spread. Lard, rancid pork fat, **goose fat**, sheep fat, and unsalted butter were commonly saved and used as healing agents. In northern areas where hunting or trapping was more common, bear and badger fat was collected and processed for medicinal uses. Wild animal fats could also be obtained from Aboriginal people, who regularly migrated through the settlement districts. Wider healing uses of wild animal fats may have been influenced by knowledge gained from Native healers. An unusual type of healing fat, reputably very effective, was dog fat *(salo vid sobaky)*. In the Old Country it was available from the village dogcatcher, who would process it from the stray animals caught. Dog fat use was not commonly described in Canada, probably because dogs were kept as pets and typically not considered nuisance animals.

Goose fat, unsalted butter, and lard were the most frequently used healing fats. They were used to not only warm up injured and painful areas but were also applied to keep rough and chapped skin soft and pliable. Fats were also taken internally, in various hot liquids, most commonly in hot milk. Fats were used in their natural state but they did not store well, especially in warm weather. If a certain type of fat was required for a specific health problem, generally someone in the neighbourhood would have it and make it available.

> *I was told that the best way to treat chapped hands* (ruky) *or feet* (nohy) *was to rub on warmed-up sheep fat* (salo vid vivtsi). *It was to be warmed up enough to be soft, but it should not be a liquid. I told this to a woman whose hands were badly chapped, and after using it for a week she was amazed as to how well her hands had healed.* — M. S. / Vegreville

## TONICS

These are typically natural products that tone the body by improving its general health and make it more resistant to illnesses. Some are also believed to be capable of cleaning the body of toxins and enhancing overall well-being. A tonic can be a simple (honey) or complex (sulphur and molasses) product or a treatment (steam bath). Its active ingredient might be a general material, such as chamomile to create a feeling of well-being, or more specific in nature, such as wormwood for toning the digestive system and liver. A tonic might be used daily, such as a shot glass of wormwood infusion; weekly, such as a steam bath; or seasonally, such as a sulphur and molasses mixture, which was considered a spring inner cleansing treatment. A consumed tonic was usually taken first thing in the morning and last thing at night or, better yet, on an empty stomach before each main meal. The portion given to children was usually one quarter to one half the dose used by an adult.

To the early Ukrainian settlers, with their limited and bland diet, tonics were an important health supplement that provided much-needed vitamins and minerals. Their crowded living conditions and poor sanitation favoured the spread of common illnesses. Taking tonics regularly was seen as an easy way to strengthen the body's resistance to such health problems.

Non-consumed plant materials were indirectly used in tonic-like applications to purify the indoor air, create a healthier household environment, or to sanitize a room with a bedridden sick individual. In a home with a sick family member, ropes of garlic were often hung on the walls, and chopped onion was scattered on the floors and windowsills. It was believed that these strong odours purified the air and killed the agents causing the illness.

Commonly used Ukrainian tonics were of two types:

## General Tonics:

These were non-specific in their application and used primarily to improve and maintain general health. They were taken to cleanse and strengthen the body or to assist it in its natural healing processes by reducing body fatigue and weakness. These were used on a regular basis and included:

*Eating:*
- two to three cloves of **garlic** or onions, with oil and sour cream / small quantities of honey / cottage cheese / grated horseradish root / sauerkraut / fresh or cooked strawberries or raspberries / shredded cabbage boiled in milk / cabbage core / boiled pigeon meat / mint heated in cow's milk / curdled milk products / 1-2 tsp. kerosene on 1 tsp. sugar.

*Drinking:* 2 3 times daily, mainly before meals, any of the following.
- Infusion of **chamomile** *(romashka),* **rosehips** *(shypshyna),* petals, or buds / dilute (1 tbsp. or shot glass in a cup of water) wormwood tops / yarrow leaves / nettle leaves / dilute or concentrated (boiled down to 10 per cent of its volume) birch sap / **raspberry leaves** *(lystky vid malyny)* or cane tips / dandelion flowers (for children) / linden flowers / mint leaves / parsley leaves / lamb's quarters tops / feverfew leaves / a mixture of chamomile flowers, feverfew leaves, rosehips and petals / a mixture of alfalfa or chamomile flowers, dried strawberries and rose petals.
- Fruit juice made from raspberry / high- or lowbush cranberry / rhubarb / blueberry.
- Decoction of couch grass rhizomes / lovage root / juniper berries / Seneca root / hawthorn fruit.
- Tincture (1 tbsp. in a cup of hot water) of elecampane roots / juniper berries.

Used on a more irregular basis were:

*Drinking:*
- equal proportions of molasses and sulphur in a cup of hot water (common spring tonic for children) / warm whey / a shot glass of wine or spirits (moonshine was preferred) with a bit of black pepper (adult males) and generally taken first thing in the morning / 1 tsp. or less of red liniment in a cup of hot water (sweetened with honey for children) / goat's milk (child) / sour milk or buttermilk (adult) / sauerkraut or pickle juice.

*Applying:*
- Rubbing Watkins or Rawleigh liniment on the body / kerosene on the soles of the feet.
- Steam bath taken weekly, using herbs, and primarily for the elderly or those with chronic aches and pains.
- Inhaling snuff or tobacco to induce sneezing (adult males).

## *Specific Tonics:*

These were used to improve the vitality of a specific organ and organ system or to prevent a specific health condition.

### STOMACH AND DIGESTIVE SYSTEM
*Eating:*
- 1 tsp. flax twice a day / dill pickle regularly.

*Drinking:*
- on a weekly basis, 1 tbsp. Epsom salts in a cup of hot water / sauerkraut juice regularly.

### KIDNEYS AND BLADDER
*Drinking:*
- whey solution, when available, regularly / infusion of rosehips, petals, or buds / a decoction of beets / a decoction of birch leaves or bark.

*Eating:*

- cooked beets.

## LIVER AND PANCREAS
*Drinking:*

- a decoction of dandelion root / an infusion of dandelion leaves.

## ARTHRITIS AND RHEUMATISM
*Eating:*

- cranberries / blueberries / rosehips.

## BRONCHITIS
*Eating:*

- 3 tbsp. crushed garlic.

## Blood Purifiers and Enhancers

Folk medicine paid particular attention to the condition of a person's blood, and therefore poor health was commonly attributed to the presence of "bad" blood. Blood's consistency was also a major concern, and efforts were made to ensure that it remained relatively thin and fluid. A number of treatments were regularly used to promote healthy blood, and these included:

*Applying:*

- cups (wet or dry) or leeches to remove "bad" blood.

*Eating:*

- garlic / onions / beets / rhubarb / chokecherries / raw or cooked peas.

*Drinking:*

- an infusion of parsley tops / yarrow leaves / wormwood tops / nettle leaves / alfalfa flowers / dill tops.
- juice of blueberries / beets.
- tincture of elecampane roots / wormwood.

- equal portions (1 tsp. for children and 1 tbsp. for adults) of molasses and sulphur in a cup of warm water.

# TEN

# Conditions Treated With Home Remedies

A wide range of the more common and non-life-threatening health problems were dealt with on a regular basis by the early Ukrainian settlers. Traditional home, or folk, remedies and treatments used commonly available resources or ones easily obtained from neighbours. The remedies were simple in nature, consisting of no more than a few ingredients, easy and quick to prepare, and easily used on a regular basis until the condition improved. When one remedy or treatment proved ineffective, another might be tried on the recommendation of someone who knew of an alternative folk treatment. When all else failed, the last resort was to pray and hope for God's grace through divine intervention. Many were healed by kitchen medicine, but many, with more serious conditions, could not be helped by such treatments. More and more, people turned to conventional medicine for their health care needs, and gradually most traditional Ukrainian folk medicine became nothing more than a historical curiosity.

The healing treatments described in this chapter are a historical record of human resourcefulness and self-reliance. They were used with considerable success because they had been formulated and tested over the centuries, and passed on from one generation to the next. Most were provided by the household matriarchs—the mother or grandmother—but a few required the involvement of specialized folk healers.

The conditions treated with traditional home remedies are described in general terms, and the remedies or treatments have been reduced to three categories: Drinking, Eating, and Applying. Most often informants were unable to provide specific details as to ingredient amounts used or details of their preparation. Also, time has clouded memories, and in many cases these descriptions are based on childhood recollections. This in no way diminishes the value of what has been shared, but it introduces a cautionary understanding that this knowledge may be incomplete. Amazingly, kitchen medicine dispensed by Baba was able to do much for the families of the early Ukrainian settlers in western Canada.


## ACHES AND PAINS

Body aches and pains were common and constant reminders of the strenuous physical work that was part of the settlers' daily life. Severe and enduring pain in the back, shoulders, neck, legs, feet, arms, and hands was not uncommon in both men and women. Heavy and improper lifting took a severe toll on the body, and not resting such injuries only prolonged and aggravated them. Seasonal chilling of exposed or poorly protected body parts was also considered to be a major source of chronic aches and pains. "Bad" blood, evidenced by swelling or bruising of the affected area, was also believed to cause aches and pains. In the elderly, these chronic aches and pains were probably due to rheumatoid arthritis, which was a painful and permanent condition. Lower back pain might also have been a sign of kidney ailment or injury. Walking and working barefoot, a common practice in the early settlement days, also contributed to swollen and aching feet.

Rest, which would have been the best remedy for such aches and pains, was impractical because of the seemingly endless daily chores. It was therefore necessary to just live with, and through, such pain until it seemed to be a "normal" body condition. More severe and disabling muscular pains that limited or prevented working were treated mainly with heat or body manipulation. Such treatments relaxed and loosened the affected muscles, often providing immediate, though not necessarily lasting, relief. Home-based treatments varied, depending on the type of pain and the body parts affected.


## General

The most common form of relief was to massage the affected areas with patent medicines such as Watkins or Rawleigh ointments and liniments / Sloan's

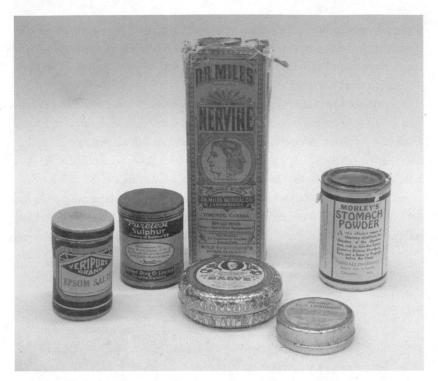

Patent medicines were available from travelling salesmen or the Eaton's catalogue. [M. MUCZ]

Liniment / oil of wintergreen / green ointment / red salve / or capsellina ointment. Household items that were similarly used included **goose fat** / wild waterfowl fat / unsalted butter / any available vegetable oil / pure vinegar / spirits / crushed garlic / or grated horseradish. These latter two preparations left an awful odour on the skin and were most often used by the elderly whose sense of smell was highly diminished and to whom pain relief was more important than the odour of the treatment. Mashed fresh nettles could also be rubbed onto painful areas for relatively immediate relief.

Paste-like homemade ointments were made from equal portions of the following ingredients: a spruce or pine gum + honey + egg yolk mixture / Vaseline + dry mustard / pine or spruce gum + lard or goose fat. Liquid liniments were made from a decoction of birchbark in a small amount of vinegar / a tincture of spruce or pine needles and dry red peppers / or a tincture of horseradish. Warm poultices, applied to affected areas overnight, consisted of potatoes, sliced into quarter-inch-thick pieces or grated / crushed burdock leaves / crushed yarrow leaves / a mustard plaster / a mixture of crushed wormwood leaves and egg white / or grated horseradish root.

Steam baths / wet or dry **cups** / leeches / dry or moist hot packs / and Epsom salts solution compresses were also used. It was considered helpful to have a drink of wormwood infusion / a comfrey leaf and root decoction / or cucumber juice. Eating crushed garlic, on bread covered with a thick layer of bacon fat, was believed to provide internal heating and help in pain relief.

More intensive body massage was not frequently used, because people did not know how to do it properly. Such a procedure required a trained specialist, and these were typically available only in cities. When such massage was done, it was mainly used on women who suffered strained abdominal muscles from improper or excessively heavy lifting. This treatment was available only if an elderly woman *(baba)* who knew how to do the procedure resided in the area.

*I strained my stomach area carrying a heavy pail of plastering clay. The area became swollen and painful, but all the doctor would suggest was that I go on a diet. I went to see a woman in our area who said she could help me. After examining me she said I was very swollen inside, but that she could treat me. She came to my place and went to the barn to collect hay* (sino) *screenings that contained different plants [healing herbs?]. She placed these in a small barrel* (bochka), *added water, and put a heated rock in. I sat, covered with a blanket, over the barrel and steamed myself. After this, she carefully but firmly massaged my abdomen for a time and had me go to bed for added rest. She repeated this treatment three evenings in a row and told me that I was not to lift anything for six weeks. I offered her money* (hroshi), *but she would not take it. In a month I was completely recovered.* — H. J. / Vegreville

## Back

Such pains, which greatly limited body movement and the possibility of doing any work, were treated with wet or dry **cups** / leeches / hot packs / steam baths /

or soaking in a tub of hot water. Often the hot bath contained a decoction of oak bark / nettles / or horseradish root. A similar soaking in a warm infusion of thyme, sage, mullein, and chamomile was also considered helpful.

> *When people got very chilled* (zastudylysia), *then leeches* (p'iavky) *were applied to their sore back. My brother got chilled once and had to have a couple of these treatments. Leeches were placed on his back, and after they had filled up on the chilled blood they fell off. This remedy helped a lot of people.*
> — N. B. / Edmonton

Manipulation of the back muscles, to loosen tightness, was also used. This was done by having the person with the sore back lie flat on their stomach, on the ground. A small child was then required to carefully walk back and forth on the back for approximately ten minutes. Another method, which required the involvement of a strong adult, involved grabbing the disabled person by their shoulders, and vigorously shaking them. Having the affected individual vigorously roll around on the ground also helped to loosen tight, sore muscles.

Massage was the most gentle and effective method of loosening up painful muscles. It involved rubbing a fatty material such as vegetable oil / unsalted butter / or lard into the painful areas. An infusion of wormwood with a tablespoon of dry mustard / or chamomile could also be rubbed in. Some individuals massaged the body with pure vinegar or a mixture of soap and alcohol. Store-bought medicinal ointments and liniments were probably the most effective materials to use because they contained ingredients that produced tissue heating and more immediate and longer-lasting relief.

Poultices were also applied to the sore area at night. These were made of nettle leaves or a paste of grated horseradish root and flour, but the skin was first covered with cream or butter to prevent blistering. A mustard plaster could also be used to quickly heat the area and provide enough relief for the sufferer to fall asleep, but these had to be used carefully because they could produce burns.

A few individuals believed that eating cooked parsnip roots and drinking a parsley infusion or a flax-seed decoction was helpful.

## Feet and Hands

Poultices were the most commonly used forms of relief for limb pain. These were applied overnight to the soles of the feet and were made from mashed wormwood foliage / moistened coltsfoot leaves / fresh or heated cabbage leaves / cut-up onions / plantain leaves / or heated and softened centre "veins" from **horseradish** *(khrin)* leaves. Hot, dry, or moist nettle infusion compresses were also used. Rubbing these painful areas with purchased ointments or liniments / unsalted butter / or with hemp oil was also widely done.

A fifteen-minute soak in a hot decoction, reheated when it had cooled, of juniper branches and berries or an infusion of nettle / chamomile / colts-foot / yarrow / nodding thistle / or a mixture of comfrey and yarrow was also an effective treatment. Sometimes the limbs were only soaked in hot water to which a tablespoon of dry mustard was added, or a hot salt solution was used. Soaking sore limbs in a solution of kerosene and warm water was smelly but helpful. Walking barefoot through a patch of nettles, handling nettles, or beating the painful limb with fresh nettles was a treatment of last resort used only by the brave and hardy who were in too much pain to consider anything less extreme.

The elderly, if beehives were available, let the bees sting their sore hands. Such extreme treatment was probably used for their constant rheumatoid arthritis pain. Placing two tablespoons of kerosene in cloth gloves and soaking these in hot water was another way to provide temporary relief for aching hands. A less commonly used remedy involved washing and heating egg-sized potatoes, placing them in the painful hand, and binding the clenched fist with a cloth wrapping. The hand was kept bound this way overnight, and the stretching may helped bring a degree of movement to the joint and some relief after the binding was removed. Cups and **leeches** were also used if the limb pain was considered to result from an accumulation of "bad" blood in the area. Bloodletting was a common practice for reducing the puffiness of swollen hands or feet.

> *Wormwood* (polyn) *is good for treating foot problems such as paralysis and gangrene sores. My brother had cancer and was losing the use of his feet* (nohy). *He received radiation treatment, but was told that he might need to have his*

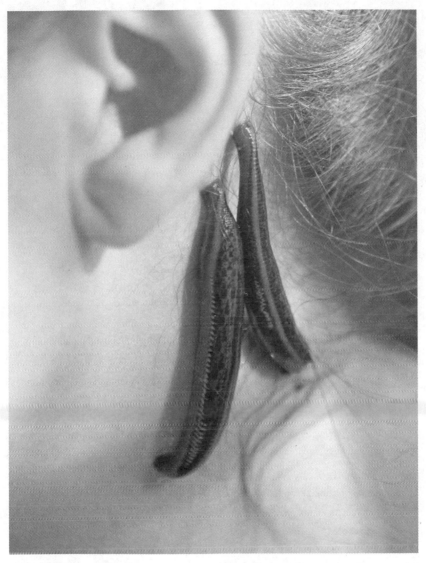

Leeches were also used to remove "bad" blood. [PHOTO COURTESY PIXMAC]

*legs amputated* (vidtynaty). *After going home, he began soaking his feet in a solution of boiled wormwood. After a few weeks he was able to move around using only a walker for support.* — E. K. / Edmonton

## ANXIETY AND NERVOUSNESS

Hard physical work with daily exposure to fresh air meant that most people fell asleep easily and slept well. Infants, young children, the ill, and distressed adults were more inclined to be restless and unable to sleep. Nervousness or persistent feelings of anxiety were uncommon, but when they did occur the affected person was typically taken to a local *baba* who knew how to pour wax (a traditional spiritual healing practice). Such severely or chronically restless individuals were thought to be possessed and required a more spiritual cure.

Restlessness and anxiety were treated with a variety of household remedies. These included:

*Drinking:*
- *Infusion* (**honey** or sugar was added for children) of **chamomile** / buttercup flowers / ginger root / mint (wild or domesticated) / hemp root or seeds / yarrow / thyme / ginseng / rosehips / wormwood / nettle / regular tea.
- half a plug of tobacco placed in a cup of tea, which produced a deep sleep.
- a cup of warm milk with 1 tsp. unsalted butter / crushed garlic in a cup of boiled milk / a few tsp. **poppy** infusion in milk (child) or water (adult), which produced a state of deep relaxation and sleep.
- small portions of a wine-based basil-leaf tincture / a shot glass (adult) or a few tbsp. (older child) or tsp. or drops (younger child) of spirits (homebrew preferred).
- a cup of boiled water in which dark salt (purchased in chunks at the store) was dissolved.
- vegetable (potato / carrot / parsley / or other available fresh vegetable) broth given to children before going to bed.

*Eating:*
- raw onions before going to bed.

*Applying:*
- *Infusion,* before going to bed, of chamomile / dry straw in a hot bath.

- placing a hot pack to the neck, shoulders, or back.
- sleeping on a pillow stuffed with fragrant hops / meadow rue.
- placing dried and crumbled wormwood shoots in a cloth sachet and wrapping in a cloth which is then put on the forehead or onto both sides of the head.
- massaging Watkins or Rawleigh camphorated ointment on a baby's belly (rubbing may also help in releasing intestinal gas and touching provides additional comfort).

## ARTHRITIS AND RHEUMATISM

Arthritis is a painful condition associated with joint inflammation. Symptoms include swelling, warmth, and reddening of the skin over the joints. Pain and restricted movement of affected hands, arms, legs, and feet occurs in its later stages. The condition produces general fatigue and sleeping difficulties. Damage to the heart, lungs, eyes, nerves, and muscles is also common. Arthritis commonly develops in people over forty and is more common in women than in men.

Rheumatism, a more varied condition of the muscles, bones, and joints, is also accompanied by pain and disability. Rheumatoid arthritis is a common condition in the elderly and produces gnarled and misshapen hands and feet. Osteoarthritis, another arthritic form, is associated with normal "wear and tear" on joints, which also leads to deterioration and chronic pain.

Collectively these muscle and joint pains are termed rheumatoid arthritis and were one of the most common afflictions of the elderly. In the old days conventional medicine knew little about these diseases and had few effective treatments. The most common medical advice was to keep the inflamed and painful joints as warm as possible. This meant that many elderly people dressed in heavy or layered clothing and wore their felt boots *(choboty)* throughout the year.

Some believed that the arthritic condition was due to chilled or "bad" blood, which could be managed with cups and/or leeches (described in chapter eight). Many elderly people also sought heating relief by sleeping on top of the indoor clay oven  or by climbing into a still-warm outdoor clay bake oven. Another widely used therapy was regularly taking a steam baths (also described in chapter eight), followed by a vigorous rubbing and massaging of

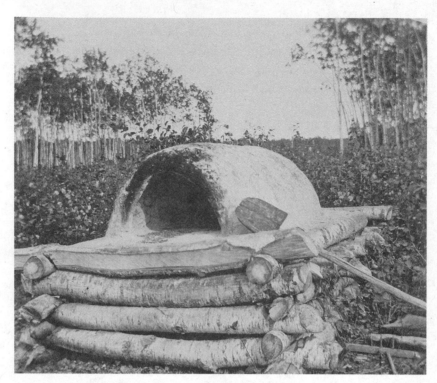
Heat from a clay oven cooked food and provided relief from arthritic pain. [PAM N9601]

the affected areas with goose fat / skunk fat / bear grease / vinegar / spirits / Watkins or Rawleigh ointments / a mixture of garlic and sulphur / a mixture of chimney soot and lard or old (rancid?) pork fat / a horseradish paste / or a fern rhizome tincture.

> *My husband's grandmother (baba) had bad arthritis, which caused her knees to swell up and hurt. She bought a bloodsucker and placed it on the swollen knee. The leech moved around on the knee (kolino), soon attached itself, and started feeding. When it was full of blood it released itself from the skin. She took it in her palm (dolonia) and squeezed it until all the blood came out. It was placed in a jar of water and could be used over and over again.* — H. S. / Chipman

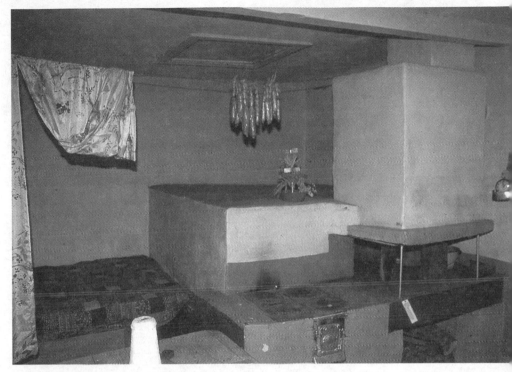

A sleeping area (top corner) on the indoor clay oven was reserved for the elderly. [M. MUCZ]

Painful joints were also soaked in hot water solutions containing hay / grass / a mixture of wildflowers / nettle leaves and/or roots / fresh or dry wormwood shoots / comfrey leaves / oats / or Epsom salts.

Some individuals washed their arthritic joints with cold water at the start of the day, which helped numb the pain. The area was then vigorously rubbed to increase blood flow, and this action did provide a short period of relief. Beating or rubbing the painful area with nettle leaves was also a common practice, since the nettle also produced a numbing effect.

*Indians* (andiiany) *came to an alkaline lake in our area and collected the whitish salts that dried up on the shore* (bereh). *They dissolved these salts in warm*

*water and soaked their arthritic feet in the solution. The local Ukrainians copied*
*this treatment.* — E. L. / Two Hills

Certain drinks and foods were also believed to assist in alleviating rheuma-toid arthritic pain, and these included:

### Drinking:
- *Infusion,* taken 3 times daily, generally before the main meal, of yarrow tops / raspberry leaves / comfrey roots and leaves / **nettle** *(kropyva)* leaves and flowers (summer) and roots (winter) / chamomile flowers / strawberry leaves (middle leaf harvested before the fruit formed) / dandelion leaves / couch grass / Seneca root / Canada or sow thistle shoots.
- liquid collected from boiled flax seeds.
- a shot glass of alcohol / homebrew.
- 1 tsp. garlic tincture.

### Eating:
- fresh parsley or radishes.
- *berries:* high- or lowbush cranberries / rosehips / blueberries.
- garlic cloves or mashed garlic mixed with 1 tsp. vinegar.

Eating fruit was also considered to be a preventative measure.

## BREAKS AND SPRAINS

Broken bones, dislocations, sprains, and crushed fingers and toes were common on the farm, where labour-intensive work often involved dangerous equipment and large animals. Serious (15 per cent of cases) injuries of this nature—multiple breaks, or those with bones protruding through the skin—were almost always taken to a medical doctor for treatment. Some minor injur-ies (25 per cent)—clean breaks, fractures, or sprains—were usually treated at home. Basic home treatment consisted of binding the injured area with

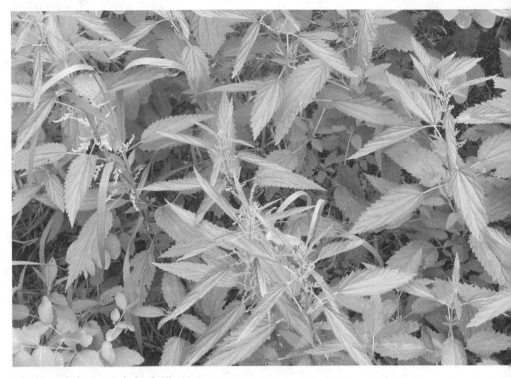
Stinging nettle leaves numbed arthritic pain. [M. MUCZ]

splints (boards) and cloth, which stabilized the injury. In many cases, self-treatment of a serious injury was not done properly and resulted in injured bones healing poorly, shortened, or slightly crooked. This could leave the person crippled for life.

*My father was a self-taught bonesetter. He was able to treat broken bones, sprains, and dislocations. He had his own homemade salve (mast) that he applied to sprains, which he then bound to keep them stable. Broken bones were set, splinted with flat boards, and then wrapped with cloth. He suggested resting such injuries until they got better. People came from all over for his help. I once awoke with a dislocated neck (shyia) that caused me severe pain. He took my neck and gently moved it back into place. He was a wonderful man.* — M. D. / Camrose

The majority (60 per cent) of skeletal injuries were treated by the local bonesetter (described in chapter four). Typical treatment involved soaking the injured area for an hour in warm whey or an Epsom salts solution, which reduced the swelling. The break was then set by gentle manipulation and it was stabilized with wooden splints, which in many cases had been brought from the Old Country. Splints could also be made from white poplar wood, but even slabs of bark, which were lighter, could be used. The splinted area was then wrapped with strips of linen cloth or hemp rope, and a sling might be made to provide additional support. Crutches, if necessary, were made from thick Y-shaped tree branches to provide support for mobility. These reduced pressure on the limb and permitted faster healing. Crushed fingers or toes were serious injuries for which doctors often recommended amputation. Most often people wanted to keep their digits and tried home remedies, which were quite successful. A traditional treatment was to soak the digits in a warm birchbark infusion; apply a salve made from beeswax, honey and spruce gum; and then bandage the injury with cloth strips. The procedure was initially repeated two to three times a day until there were signs of healing, after which the treatment was administered only once daily.

Children born or afflicted with crippled limbs were, out of desperation, also treated with various home remedies. Daily bathing of the crippled limbs in an infusion of young birch twigs or wormwood was followed by massaging the limbs. Such simple treatment provided some physical improvement and undoubtedly emotional comfort and support to both child and parent. It provided the child with hope that his or her condition would and could improve. An extreme home remedy for treating crippled feet was to have the child drink an infusion of pig manure. Its effectiveness, if any, was never confirmed, but its use may have been based on an association with the strength and sturdiness of a pig's limbs.

*My younger brother developed a terrible condition [polio?], which produced painful cramping and twisting in different parts of his body. Mother bathed him, four to five times a day, in a warm (teplyi) solution made by boiling young birch leaves (lystia vid berezy). This condition caused many children in our area to die, but my mother saved my brother.* — C. O. / Edmonton

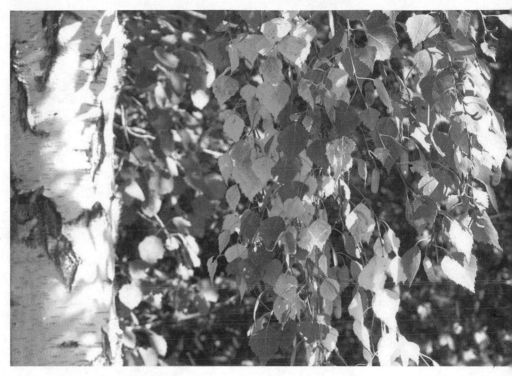

Birch leaf and branch solutions provided relief to crippled limbs.
[PHOTO COURTESY PUBLIC-DOMAIN-IMAGE.COM]

## CIRCULATORY PROBLEMS

Heart and blood circulation conditions were poorly understood by both folk and conventional medical practitioners in the early days. Folk remedies relied heavily on the principles associated with the Doctrine of Signatures, which viewed similarly coloured or shaped plant parts as being useful in treating corresponding body structures or systems. Red-coloured plant materials would therefore be most useful in dealing with problems related to the heart and blood circulation. It was also widely believed that "bad" blood, which was thick, dark, and congested, contributed to a number of body ills. Chronic, deep, and aching pains were considered to be symptoms of such blood accumulation or "pooling" in different body parts. To treat these conditions it was necessary to remove such blood by means of leeches or wet cupping. Similarly, chronic hand and foot puffiness was thought to indicate high blood pressure, and this could also be reduced by regulated bloodletting.

Excessive and frequent consumption of alcohol was considered to be bad for the circulation and the heart. Heavy drinking caused facial flushing and a network of fine surface blood vessels to form on the nose, evidence that alcohol affected the circulatory system.

Home-based practices to deal with the heart and circulatory system were typically more preventative than curative. These were used on a relatively regular basis, mainly by adults or the elderly. Remedies were generally taken, for maximum effect, first thing in the morning or on an empty stomach before a meal, often three times a day.

## HIGH BLOOD PRESSURE

This could be most easily reduced or controlled with bloodletting, using leeches or wet cupping. Garlic, considered to be highly effective in keeping blood pressure down, was also a common ingredient in Ukrainian home remedies for circulatory problems. Onions, however, were considered to elevate blood pressure and were not commonly used in treating such conditions.

Common treatments included:

*Drinking:*
- *Infusion* of parsley tops / mint leaves / wormwood tops (1 tbsp. or half a shot glass full-strength, or diluted in a hot drink or water) / yarrow tops / rose petals / nettle tops / chamomile flowers.
- *Decoction* of birch / white poplar (aspen) / cabbage leaves.
- juice made from a whole lemon, added to hot sugar water.
- mixture, 1 tbsp. taken daily, of two mashed garlic cloves, juice of 2–3 lemons, and a half cup of honey, all added to a cup of hot water.

*Eating:*
- 1 or 2 cloves of garlic / grated horseradish root / cooked rhubarb / raspberries (fresh or cooked) / cooked beets.

## HEART PROBLEMS

Keeping the heart fit was typically not a major concern, because people had daily exercise in walking long distances and were involved in considerable physical labour. A weak heart, however, was believed to be strengthened by:

### Drinking:
- *Infusion* of chamomile flowers / mint leaves / wormwood tops / parsley leaves / rose petals.
- *Decoction* of parsnip roots / spruce gum.
- cranberry juice with half a shot glass of alcohol.
- **goat's milk** *(moloko vid kozy)*.

> *Anyone who had a heart problem was told to take a shot of homebrew and hope that the problem would pass. Waiting for it to pass, they would often just go outside for some fresh air* (povitria), *because this was all they could do at the time. Many died doing this. It would have been so much better to get them to a doctor as quickly as possible, but this was impossible in the early years* (pershi roky). — M. M. / Vegreville

### Eating:
- on a daily basis: 1 or 2 cloves of raw garlic / onions / strawberries.

## COLDS AND FLU

These two seasonal—winter and early spring—illnesses were a common health problem for the early settlers and revealed the greatest number and variety of home-based remedies. Both were highly contagious viral respiratory infections (unknown as such even by the doctors of the time) and spread quickly in the crowded homestead household. Children were especially vulnerable because of their underdeveloped immune systems, and therefore a cold or the flu quickly spread throughout the family.

A cold developed slowly and produced a headache, low fever, sore throat, nasal and chest congestion, a runny nose, and breathing difficulties. It occurred more frequently than the flu, was shorter in duration, and was also less severe. It incubated over a two- to three-day period after initial infection, and typically lasted about three days. It would often clear up on its own in about a week. Individuals were contagious only as long as they showed symptoms.

Influenza (the flu) was a less-common but more serious illness. It developed quickly and caused a dry cough, fever, and fatigue associated with general body aches. The danger of the flu was that it could worsen and lead to more severe health problems, such as bronchitis or pneumonia. This was a concern, especially for the very young and the elderly. Once caught, it lasted from a few days to a couple of weeks, depending on an individual's age and stamina. It started with a sore throat, but quickly escalated into a high fever, severe chills, a bad headache that could lead to delirium, severe muscle and joint aches, and overall fatigue and weakness. There was less nasal congestion than in a cold, but it would result in a dry hacking cough. Flu, varying in its severity from year to year, had the potential to develop into a local epidemic or into a rarer global pandemic.

The Spanish flu pandemic of October 1918 through March 1919 had a devastating global effect. It was calculated that it resulted in 20 to 25 million deaths worldwide. Its severity was evidenced by its symptoms developing in as little as twelve to fourteen hours after infection, and it affected healthy young adults as well as children and the elderly. Once infected, most of these young adults recovered slowly and poorly or died unexpectedly. There have been suggestions that this vulnerability, in seemingly healthy young people, may have been associated with undiagnosed tuberculosis bacteria that the individuals may have carried. Although the individuals did not show sign of tuberculosis, their respiratory systems would have been weakened and thus more affected by the flu virus.

*My parents went into town* (misto) *for supplies and caught the Spanish flu. Soon we were all sick, and the kids developed bad nose bleeds. Dad, although sick himself, looked after all six of us and would boil milk with bread dough to feed us. Dad was sick for over a year and a half and had to be hospitalized for a while. When he came home, Mother had a man come and apply cups* (banky) *to dad's aching back. These treatments did provide him some relief.* — O. A. / Lamont

It became quickly evident that in households where garlic and homebrew were regularly used, there were fewer and less severe incidences of the flu. This association was identified for Ukrainian bloc settlement areas and doctors recognized the importance of these materials in dealing with the flu. In many Ukrainian households, baskets of garlic were distributed throughout the house and cut onions were placed on windows sills to ward off infection. Discoloration of the onions was taken as a sign that they were doing their job. The demand for garlic became so widespread that its price in some areas increased to as much as $1 per pound, which was a significant amount of money at that time. Non-Ukrainians commonly visited Ukrainian settlement areas with the hope of being able to buy garlic and, undoubtedly, some homebrew as well.

*Our family did not get sick during the flu* (hryp) *epidemic of 1918 because we always ate a lot of garlic. Our neighbours had the flu, and we looked after their livestock for them when they were sick. A local half-breed [Métis?] family had seven people dead* (mertvi) *in their house at one time. It was terrible—so many people died from it.* — S. S. / Mundare

A widely used preventative practice during the Spanish flu pandemic was to identify affected individuals or families and quarantine them at home. Local health and public officials closed down schools, churches, and public buildings. Holding of public meetings, weddings, and funerals was greatly restricted. For funerals, often only the priest, the immediate family, and a few relatives were present. People were discouraged from going out and socializing for fear of spreading the flu. Individuals who went into town for supplies had to wear layered gauze facemasks. In some cases the store's goods were displayed on tables outside the building to minimize the flu's spread. Families whose normally able-bodied adults were ill depended on the generosity of their neighbours to look after essential farm chores, such as feeding and watering the farm animals. Often a healthy or less-sick individual would spend the morning doing their own chores and then spend the rest of the day doing farm chores for ailing neighbours. Firewood and drinking water were essentials for the household and, since the ill had little appetite, an adequate supply of drinking water and wood

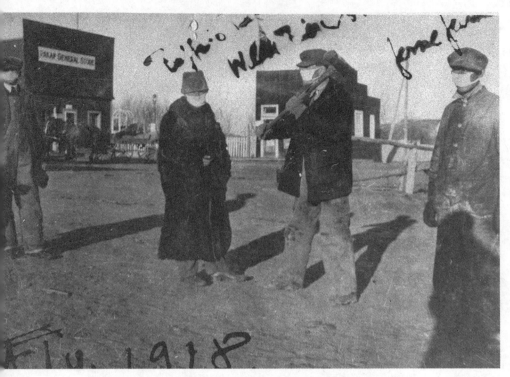

Cloth masks provided protection during the 1918–1919 flu pandemic. [PAA UV6]

was their main concern. These items were left outside the door so the flu "bug" was not spread to the healthy visitor. In some hard-hit areas without a hospital, schools were converted to accommodate and treat the sick. Ill people were looked after by volunteers and treated by the local doctor. The lack of a hospital and medical services in many remote rural areas meant that flu mortality rates were much higher.

> *Five in our family had the flu, and only my mother and brother were healthy enough to get what supplies (postachannia) we needed from town. The supplies were dropped off two miles from town so that people from homes with the flu would not have to come into town and infect others. Many people were dying everywhere.* — P. M. / Mundare

Colds and flu show similar symptoms, especially in their early stages, and were often called by one term or the other, depending on their severity. Because of this misidentification, they both were treated in much the same way and with similar home remedies. Staying well-covered in bed or sitting, while fully clothed and covered with blankets, near a stove was the most common treatment. Additionally, various products and treatments, differing somewhat for children and adults, were used to deal with the conditions the illnesses produced. Fluid intake was seen as important, so most of the remedies were taken in liquid form. Loss of appetite also restricted the treatments that required ingredients to be eaten.

> *During the 1918–1919 flu epidemic, people were told to stay at home* (perebuvaty vdoma) *so that they would not catch or spread the flu. My father protected himself from it by drinking homebrew each morning and eating garlic* (chasnyk) *throughout the day. He went all over the place, helping neighbours who were sick or dying, but he never caught the flu.* — W. S. / Chipman

In the treatments listed below, an indication is given as to whether the remedy was suggested as being used primarily for colds (C), the flu (F), or either (C/F) illness. Home remedies and treatments included.

### Applying:

- *Salve or paste* of crushed garlic (a child's delicate skin was first coated with a protective layer of goose fat) (C/F) / **goose fat** / chicken fat / lard or unsalted butter, which was applied directly, or on paper, to the body (C) / bear fat (C) / a mixture of equal parts goose fat and turpentine (C) / a mixture of mashed garlic, vinegar, camphor oil, and alcohol (F) / crushed garlic and horseradish mixed with honey (C/F) / crushed garlic, vegetable oil, and a bit of sulphur (F) / Watkins or Rawleigh liniment (C) / or a mixture of crushed garlic and onions (child) (C). The various materials were rubbed on the chest, upper back, neck, soles of the feet, and the inner wrists. The person had to keep warm by remaining well clothed, staying by the oven or stove, or going to bed and being wrapped with flannel cloth or towels on the body parts treated with the home remedy.

- on the chest or back, any of the following materials: a mustard plaster (C/F) / a crushed garlic or grated horseradish poultice to the chest and a woollen sock, soaked in melted goose fat, wrapped around the throat (C) / a poultice of grated raw potatoes wrapped around the feet, hands, and forehead of babies and infants (C/F) / a boiled flax poultice on the chest (F) / a hot pack on the aching parts of the body (F) / placing a towel soaked with healthy child's urine on a sick child's forehead and giving the child plenty of boiled water to drink (F).
- *Steam bath:* containing a pine- or spruce-needle or spruce-gum infusion (C/F) to the face / full-body steam bath with an infusion of nettles and raspberry leaves (C/F).
- heating the body by being heavily dressed and covered with quilts and blankets, while sitting near a hot oven or stove. When in bed, it was necessary to remain well covered with sheets and quilts. The body was also fully rubbed down with a patent liniment (C/F) for added internal heating.
- cups (wet) to the arms or leeches to the feet (C).

*My sister's granddaughter* (vnuchka) *had a very bad cold* (paskudna zastuda), *and nothing that she was doing was helping to cure it. My sister realized there still was something else to try. She crushed up some garlic and wrapped it in a piece of cloth so that it would not burn the skin. She placed such a cloth on the sole* (pidoshva) *of each foot and the sock was pulled over to keep everything in place. The girl fell asleep and when she woke up the next morning, the cold was gone.* — M. S. / Lamont

### Drinking:
- *Fruit juices* made from **cranberry** *(kalyna)* (C) / black currant (C) / chokecherry (C) / raspberry (C/F) / or any other available fruit. 2 tbsp. of the fruit concentrate was added to a cup of hot water, and for a child, 1 tsp. or 1 tbsp. of sweetener (honey or sugar) was added to make the drink easier to take.

- *Infusion* of **chamomile** flowers (C) / **linden** *(lypa)* flowers (C) / wormwood and mint tops (C, coughs) / rose petals or hips (C, coughs) / yarrow leaves (C/F) / angelica flowers, leaves and roots (C/F) / mint leaves (C) / mullein leaves (C) / thyme leaves (C) / lilac flowers (C) / sage leaves (C) / dandelion leaves (C) / nettle leaves (C, coughs) / strawberry leaves (C) / raspberry leaves (C) / or hemp leaves (C/F). These teas were taken 3 times daily, and honey or sugar was added to a child's drink.
- *Decoction,* 3 times daily, of ginger root (C) / parsley roots (C) / beets (C/F) / blueberry stems (C) taken by the cupful / red willow twigs (C/F, headaches and aches) / equal parts of willow and elm bark plus birch buds (C) / or pine or spruce buds (C) taken 1 tbsp. at a time.
- a cup of any hot liquid (C/F) / 1 tbsp. badger or bear fat in a cup of hot water (C/F) / a cup of hot, scalded, or diluted milk (child). Hot water was used for children, if no milk was available, and also used by adults. 1 tsp. **goose** or chicken fat, or butter, and a sweetener for children, was added to the hot liquid (C) / hot milk containing crushed and strained garlic juice or goose fat and crushed garlic, sweetened with honey for children (C/F) / 1 tsp. (child) or 1 tbsp. (adult) of Watkins or Rawleigh red liniment to which a sweetener was added for children (C) / sour milk (F) / honey in boiled milk or water (C) / fresh cow's milk (F) / hot milk with an egg beaten into it (C) / a cup of hot water, with 1 tbsp. each of lemon juice and a sweetener (child) or the juice of a whole lemon (adult) (C) / 1 tsp. kerosene in a cup of milk (C) / a cup of hot milk or water containing two chopped cloves of garlic plus 2 tbsp. **goose fat** or butter (C/F) / a shot glass of whisky every few hours (adult) / a full shot glass of a tincture made from dissolving a few tsp. burnt sugar and ½ tsp. or ½ tbsp. black pepper in a pint of whisky (C/F) / a few tbsp. or a shot glass of whisky in half a cup of hot water (adult); children were given 1 tsp. or 1 tbsp. whisky with sweetener added—this mixture would induce sweating (C/F) / 1 tsp. melted lard with a shot glass of whisky (C/F) / a cup of tea containing a shot glass of lemon juice, honey, and whisky (C/F) / a shot glass of whisky with 1 tbsp. black or cayenne pepper (C/F) / a few drops of whisky and Hoffmann's Drops on 1 tbsp. sugar (C/F) / equal parts of honey, lemon juice, and homebrew (C/F) / 1 tsp. melted

goose fat in a shot glass of whisky (C/F) / 1 tbsp. honey in a shot glass of whisky (C/F) / a few tbsp. or a shot glass of a tincture made from a few drops of poppy resin in whisky (C/F) / a shot glass of tincture made from crushed garlic in **whisky** or wine (F) / a shot glass of red liniment, garlic, and alcohol (F).

- broth of an old chicken, given to children (C/F) / cattail rhizomes, cabbage, and onions (C/F).
- 1 or 2 drops of kerosene (adult) or sweetened with 1 tsp. sugar for children (C/F, coughs).
- *Cough syrup*, used for both colds and flu and taken 3 times a day in a 1 tsp. (child) or 1 tbsp. (adult) dose. These were made from the strained liquids of boiled onions and honey or a large onion was hollowed out, filled with honey and butter, and heated in the oven until it liquefied / boiled onions / boiled raspberries sweetened with sugar / spruce and pine buds (1:2 ratio) boiled in water and sugar added / willow and elm bark plus birch buds boiled in water / a large peeled and hollowed-out beet filled with sugar and heated in the oven until it liquefied / 3-4 cloves of garlic crushed and added along with ¼ tsp. cayenne pepper to ½ cup hot lemon juice / a beaten egg sprinkled with sugar (for young children).

*Mother collected and dried rosehips. These would be boiled for a long time, then strained, and then sugar (tsukor) was added to the liquid. She used this syrup as a cough and cold remedy, but she would ration it out, a shot glass at a time. She even had to hide (khovaty) it from us kids, because we liked its taste so much that we would have even taken it when we were not sick (my ne buly slabi).*
— M. D. / Vegreville

*Eating:*
- 2 cloves of garlic washed down with a cup of hot water (C).
- garlic, taken at bed time, **crushed** *(rozdusheni)* or sliced and placed on a piece of bread thickly covered with salted bacon fat or lard (adult) or unsalted butter (child). This was washed down with a cup of warm water, sweetened with **honey** or sugar (child) (C/F) / 2 cloves taken daily

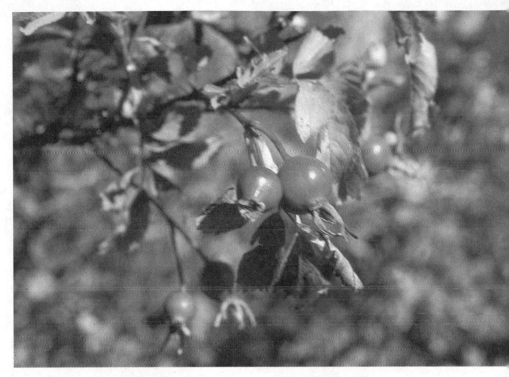

Rosehips made a cough syrup for colds and flu. [M. MUCZ]

by adults, but too hard on children's stomachs (C/F) / crushed and taken with cut-up strips of pork fat, which were eaten first to lubricate and protect the throat. The two were eaten alternately until all the garlic was gone (C) / or crushed or whole and washed down with pickle juice (C).

- boiled highbush cranberries (C).

- *Mixture* of horseradish, salt, and vinegar on a piece of bread, with the throat wrapped with an old sock soaked in melted goose fat (C) / grated radish (black or red) and honey (C) / cabbage or parsley leaves (C) / a few drops of Watkins or Rawleigh red liniment on 1 tsp. sugar (C) / a small ball of Watkins or Rawleigh ointment rolled in sugar and swallowed (C) / 1 or 2 Hoffmann's Drops in 1 tsp. sugar, which helped open the nasal passages (C) / 1 tbsp. each of goose fat and honey (C) / 1 tsp. cayenne pepper mixed with 1 tbsp. honey, which was licked slowly for maximum benefit (C).

# COLIC

A fussy baby is a major source of irritation, distraction, and concern for anyone hearing it. In most cases such distress was probably due to severe abdominal pain from the accumulation of intestinal gas. Such a problem would easily develop if the child was fed cow's milk before it was capable of digesting it, if it was allergic to cow's milk, or if it was fairly inactive and could not expel such gases naturally. Typically, a breast-fed baby does not experience gas buildup, and neither does one who is carried around or rocked in someone's arms. Any activity helps to release such gas and prevents its buildup. A colicky or fussy child disrupted its mother's work during the day and made restful sleep for the rest of the family difficult at night.

Common home remedies used to treat the problem included:

*Drinking:*
- a few drops of unripe poppy seed or pod decoction added to an infant's drink.
- 1 tbsp. **honey** or sugar, added to a cup of boiled water, and 2-3 tsp. fed to a child.
- 2-3 drops of spirits in the child's milk.
- crushed-up unripe poppy seeds and/or pods placed into a knotted cloth soother, which the child would suck on.
- a moist cloth soother with sugar in it, which the child would suck on.
- *Decoction*, a few tsp. given at a time, of boiled and strained pearl barley.
- *Infusion*, a few tsp. given at a time, of chamomile flowers / mint leaves / regular tea.

*Applying:*
- Rubbing the child, after its bath, with goose fat / sweet cream. The knees were also pressed to the opposite elbows, which massaged the digestive tract.

*My grandmother (baba) told me that in the Old Country a fussy baby was treated with poppy extract. Green poppy heads were collected and boiled in milk. Giving the baby just one tablespoon of this liquid (ridyna) was enough to keep it sleeping soundly for twenty-four hours or more. — J. S. / Lamont*

# COMMON DISEASES

Major illnesses, due to common diseases, seriously disrupted farm and household operations, especially if they affected a parent. When a mother became sick and there were no older children in the family, neighbourhood women might take the young children until she got better. In many cases they would also come and do the regular major household chores such as baking and cooking, washing, and gardening. If it was the husband who was sick, the wife would simply add many of his chores to her own workload and ask the children to do more. Physically demanding work, such as putting in or taking off the crop, would be done by male neighbours and relatives. When children became ill, especially with a contagious disease such as diphtheria, measles, or chicken pox, the family could be quarantined for as long as six to eight weeks. This caused great hardship for the family, because they could not go to town for supplies and were also prevented from socializing with friends and neighbours.

The more serious Old Country diseases, such as cholera and typhoid fever, were relatively unknown in Canada because of better sanitation and hygiene practices, as well as closer monitoring by health agencies. Serious illnesses did occur, however, and initial attempts to deal with them often used traditional household remedies. A common practice was to keep the sick person well covered in bed and in a warm dark room with the windows shut. Keeping the patient warm was considered important in helping to "sweat out" the illness. Cold, fresh air was believed to worsen the condition because prevailing thought was that many serious illnesses were spread by means of "bad vapours" in the outside air. Unfortunately, prolonged bed rest could produce its own complications, such as constipation, stiff muscles and joints, lung congestion, and blood clots.

Major illnesses that were treated with a limited range of home remedies are described below.


## Consumption (tuberculosis)

This is a contagious bacterial lung disease that is spread through coughing. It often causes the sick person to develop a fever, sweat heavily at night, experience severe coughing spells that could bring up blood, and lose weight. The most effective treatment, practised by conventional medical standards of the time, was to have the affected person rest and get plenty of fresh air and sunshine.

Traditional home treatments included:

*Drinking:*

- a cup, 3-4 times a day, of birch sap / infusions of linden flowers or violet leaves and flowers / hot milk with 1 tsp. (child) or 1 tbsp. (adult) badger fat / hot water with 1 tsp. dog fat / raw eggs / fresh cow's milk / a tincture of calamus root / strained liquid from cooked rolled oats.
- small portions of an extract of plantain leaves fermented for three weeks in honey.

*Eating:*

- a lot of garlic.

*Applying:*

- rubbing garlic on the neck and chest.
- soaking a piece of cloth in a wormwood tincture and placing it on the chest for 7-8 hours at a time.
- placing half a pail of whitewash (lime) solution near the bed and keeping the windows uncurtained but closed. Sunlight, and breathing the solution's fumes, helped the lungs clear up.

*My aunt had tuberculosis, and the doctor told her to go home, rest, and get fresh air. A neighbour told her that she could treat herself even better by drinking fresh cow's milk (svizhe moloko vid korovy). My aunt went to the barn each morning and evening (ranok i vechir) to do this. As the cows were being milked, she would collect a cup of warm, fresh milk and drink it. The milk may have helped, but getting out of the stuffy house and walking in the fresh air may also have been important. When the doctor examined her later on, he was surprised to find that she was free of TB. — E. L. / Viking*

## Diphtheria

This acute bacterial infection causes general weakness, a sore throat, and a fever. The infected throat becomes swollen and painful as bacterial toxins circulate in the blood. It was potentially lethal, especially if it made swallowing and breathing very difficult. Over time it could also seriously damage heart, nerve, and kidney tissues. This condition was a major cause of death, especially in young children, until a vaccine was developed in the 1920s. Immunization for it became common by the 1940s.

> *My infant died of diphtheria in the Old Country. He got sick and quickly developed a blistered ulcer (boliak) in his throat (horlo). This made it very difficult for him to breathe. We sent for a doctor, but he said there was nothing that he could do for him. Later on, some women told me that I should have put my finger down his throat and broken up the blisters to open up his breathing. I didn't know that there was something I could have done to save his life (zhyttia).* — N. B. / Edmonton

The condition was commonly treated with such home remedies as:

**Drinking:**
- 2 tbsp. kerosene twice a day.

**Applying:**
- brushing the inside of the throat, using a goose or rooster feather, with a mixture of whisky, lemon juice, and honey.
- mixing powdered sulphur in hot water and inhaling the vapours.
- sticking a finger into the throat and breaking up the ulcerations blocking the air passage.

> *My brother caught diphtheria, and his throat got so swollen that he could barely breathe. Mother made a mixture of alcohol, lemon juice, and honey to treat this.*

*She applied the mixture, with a goose* (huska) *or rooster* (kohut) *tail feather,*
*to the infected area on his throat* (horlo). *She repeated this treatment until his*
*throat cleared up completely.* — S. S. / Mundare

## Measles

This common and contagious viral disease mainly affects children. Before conventional medicine knew how to treat it, outbreaks of measles occurred every
two or three years throughout the country. Its victims developed a fever, runny
eyes and nose, and a sore throat with white-centred red spots on it. A blotchy red
rash would then develop on the face and spread to other parts of the body. The
condition weakened the patient and made them more vulnerable to secondary
infections, such as middle-ear infections or pneumonia, either of which could
be lethal.

The basic folk treatment was to keep the sick person indoors and confined
to a warm, dark room. The disease, if untreated, was known to produce eye problems. It was commonly believed, in Old Country folk medicine practices, that
bright light (sunshine) contributed to this and therefore it was best to keep the
person in relative darkness. Drinking mare's milk was also thought to speed
recovery. The patient could also drink infusions or fruit juices. Salty or sour foods
were restricted, and only "light," easily eaten foods, such as soups, were recommended. The skin rash was treated, three to four times a day, with goose fat / a
sulphur and goose fat mixture / or sour milk compresses.

## Chicken Pox

This is also a common and highly contagious childhood viral disease. Its symptoms are a mild fever and development of small itchy spots that initially form
on the trunk of the body and then spread to the limbs and face. The condition
remains infectious until the last spotted areas dried up and flaked off, which
occurs after about two weeks. Home treatment practices were similar to those
for measles. In addition to the similar liquids and foods used, eating strawberries was considered to be helpful. This practice may well have been associated

with the Doctrine of Signatures, in which the spots on the berry corresponded to the disease's spots on the body. This implied that the condition could be cured by using strawberries. Typically, the sores were treated to reduce itching and to induce scab formation with a minimum of scarring. This included:

*Applying:*
- covering the sores, 3-4 times daily, with sheep fat / goose fat / a mixture of sulphur and goose fat or lard / baking soda paste / cornstarch solution / Watkins or Rawleigh ointment.
- a sour milk compress / a cooked flax-seed poultice.
- bathing in a solution of baking soda and then applying Vaseline to keep the sores moist and soft.

## Diabetes

This serious hereditary illness involves the body's inability to properly process dietary sugars and results in development of abnormally high blood-sugar levels. There are two types of diabetes *(solodka krov),* one developing in younger people (juvenile diabetes) and the other in later adulthood (adult-onset diabetes). Their symptoms are excessive thirst and abnormally excessive production of urine with a high sugar content. In the old days, conventional medicine knew little about this disease and had few treatments for it. The majority of the diabetes that people developed was probably of the adult-onset type, since there was little mention of children dying from this condition. Nevertheless, it is possible that many of the sudden and unexplained early childhood deaths were due to diabetes. Often, in response to a question about cause of death, an informant responded, "Who knew *(khto znav)?*"

A number of informants indicated that the incidence of diabetes-like symptoms was much less common in areas where blueberries were frequently eaten. This might have more of a genetic, rather than a dietary, explanation, since it was the Bukovinians who settled in the more wooded areas where blueberries were more abundant.

Home remedies, though limited in number, were widely used to treat the symptoms of diabetes, and some may have also been used to prevent the condition from developing. These included:

*Drinking:*

- *Infusion,* 2-3 times a day, of blueberry leaves / yarrow shoots / parsley leaves / half (concentrated) to a full (diluted) shot glass of wormwood.
- a cup of fresh cow's milk.

> *My brother's wife* (zhinka) *was a diabetic, and the doctor's medicines were not helping her much. My brother was visiting a nearby reserve and an Indian woman told him how his wife could be helped. She told him to collect wormwood, boil a handful of it at a time, strain the liquid, and then keep the liquid in a jug* (zbanok). *His wife was to drink about half an ounce of this bitter* (hirkyi) *concentrate, two or three times a day. In two months, using the wormwood solution, she was fully cured of the sugar diabetes.* — M. K. / Smoky Lake

*Eating:*

- blueberry preserves.
- cooked rhubarb.
- whole or mashed garlic.

> *I will tell you* (ia skazhu vam), *back then no one knew anything about sugar diabetes* (solodka krov), *not even the doctors. People who ate a lot of blueberries* (chornytsi) *or drank blueberry tea did not seem to get diabetes. In the Smoky Lake area there were a lot of blueberries used, and not too many people there had sugar diabetes.* — P. N. / Lamont

## EAR PROBLEMS

Earaches occurred in both young and old, but they usually were a greater problem for children and made them highly agitated and restless. They were more common in winter, and thought to be caused by a bare head being exposed to the cold. Long periods of confinement in a stuffy, smoky house may also have been a contributing factor. Adults were able to suffer through such annoying pain, but simple home remedies were available and readily used. Treatments were effective and provided temporary relief, and most earaches cleared up naturally.

The treatments were almost always an application of some ingredient or a manipulation of the affected ear. These included:

### Applying:

- *Oil*: a few drops in the ear *(vukho)* or soaked into a piece of cotton, of light sewing machine oil / hemp oil / camphorated oil / any vegetable oil. Sometimes a bit of pepper was added to the oil.
- *Solution* of sauerkraut juice / melted honey / glycerine / melted goose fat / vinegar / warm sugar water / Watkins or Rawleigh ointment.
- piece of raw onion put into the ear, covered with a hot, moist cloth.
- to the outside of the painful ear: a cool, wet compress / slices of potato, wrapped on / a warm pack (heated grain or salt) / keeping the painful side of the head close to the stove and well covered / a warm, moist compress / placing the ear against cold and damp soil.
- *Rubbing* a garlic clove over the middle area of the outer surface of the ear / camphorated ointment on the outer surface of the ear.
- *Smoke:* from burning tobacco (**pipe** or cigarette) blown into the ear / a wax-coated cloth, used in making Easter eggs, burned in a dish and the smoke directed into the ear.
- steam, from boiling chamomile tea, directed into the ear with a paper funnel.
- gently blowing into a child's ear through cupped hands.
- waxed cotton string, or a candle wick, placed into the ear and gently pulled out. This removes compacted earwax or debris from the inner ear.
- a few drops of mother's milk, into a fussy baby's ear. This was done two or three times a day until the problem cleared up.
- an ear candle application (described in chapter eight).

*When someone in the family had an earache* (bil u vusi), *Mother would bring out the wax-and-varnish-coated rag she used for making Easter eggs* (pysanky). *She placed the soiled rag on a plate and then lit it. The sore ear was held over its smoke* (dym), *which entered the ear and helped reduce the pain.*
— M. D. / Vegreville

It was also suggested that eating cranberries, either fresh or rehydrated, both cured and prevented earaches.

## EYE PROBLEMS

Sight is a vital sense, and eye *(oko)* problems were considered to be serious developments that had to be carefully, if not medically, treated. Only the most minor problems were dealt with at home. The most common problems were eyestrain from poor lamp lighting, and eye irritation from foreign matter. The latter was a more common condition during haying and harvesting activities. Minor eye infections, due to poor hygiene, were also common. The eyes would become red, watery, or dry, and pus would crust on the edges. It was known that any cleaning of the eye had to be done with warm, boiled water to ensure that no additional infection was introduced by the treatment.

## *Sore*

Treatment involved:

*Applying:*
- gently blowing onto the sore eye(s): ground nasturtium roots / blue stone (copper sulphate) / powdered sugar, which produced tearing.
- slices of fresh potato (¼- or ½-inch slices) over the eye(s), wrapped in place.
- *Compress* wetted with cold water / human urine / an infusion of lily of the valley leaves / or regular tea, wrapped on with a piece of cloth.
- gentle bath of warm or cold boiled water by holding the cup against the eye and keeping it in place for a few minutes.
- dilute (1 tsp. per ½ cup water) boric acid solution.
- boiled egg white with the yolk removed, wrapped in place with a clean cloth and left on for at least 15 minutes.

# Debris

Treatment involved:

### Applying:

- a few grains of whole or powdered sugar onto the eye, letting the tearing reaction wash out the debris. The material was then wiped away with a clean cloth.
- *Seeds*, 1 or 2 placed under the eyelid, of **basil** *(bazylik)* / thyme / sweet william. The seed's irritation caused the eye to tear up and produce a slimy secretion that washed the debris out to the corner of the eye. The seeds and foreign material were then removed with a clean cloth.
- a long hair placed on the eye and used to pull out the debris, which would attach to the hair.
- tip of a rolled-up linen or cotton cloth, moistened with boiled water or saliva, to brush the debris out. The eye was then washed out with the remaining warm boiled water.
- tongue used to locate and remove the irritating debris. The ability to do this was considered a "gift" or talent that only a few women possessed. Their services were widely sought out and the effectiveness of their treatment widely recognized.
- washing the eye with warm boiled water to flush out the debris.
- edge of a clean silver coin, used to gently scrape off the debris. This was more easily done on an adult, who could tolerate the associated discomfort.

# Infection

Treatment involved:

### Applying:

- a puppy's tongue to lick off the pus. The licking action also stimulated blood flow to the eye and the relatively antiseptic saliva sped up healing.

- a compress, dipped in warm boiled water, and wrapped on. This was repeated 3 times daily to keep the eye from crusting over.
- mucous-like secretion, collected from the top of a relatively fresh cow dropping (preferably from a cow that is lactating).
- *Solution*, dropped on the eye, of equal portions of water and alcohol / weak salt solution, repeated 3 times daily / mother's breast milk for an infant.

*The cure for someone who was losing their eyesight (zir) was to go and collect the small amount of mucous which formed on the top of a fresh "cow-pie." This "juice" was kept in a bottle (fliashka) and was applied to the eye with the tip of the finger. This would be done a number of times.* — M. D. / Vegreville

## Styes

Treatment involved:

### Applying:
- a moist compress, dipped into a warm and weak solution of baking soda or salt or regular tea. This was kept on for five minutes.
- compress, re-warmed and re-wetted and reapplied until the stye burst. The area was washed with warm boiled water and dried with a clean cloth.

## Cataracts

Treatment involved:

### Applying:
- powdered sugar or finely ground tobacco onto the eyeball. This was left to dissolve, and the residue was scraped off with one edge of a silver coin or dull knife.

• raw egg white and blinking to spread it around. This was left on for a few minutes before it was washed off with warm boiled water.


## FATIGUE AND LETHARGY

Daily emotional and physical stress took its toll on the early settlers. Fatigue, which reduced normal functioning, was a common condition and resulted from the excessive physical demands of establishing and running a homestead. This problem was more common in women because of the greater and more varied demands placed on them, plus the compounding influence of their social isolation on remote homesteads. A number of home remedies were tried to alleviate such debilitating fatigue when it became prolonged and excessive. In many cases its roots were more emotional than physical, and such treatments were not overly effective.

Treatments included:

*Drinking:*
• boiled and strained liquid from juniper berries and branches.
• *Fruit beverage:* 2 tbsp. in a cup of hot water of cranberry / raspberry / pin cherry juice.
• pickle or sauerkraut juice.
• *Infusion* of chamomile / wormwood / a mixture of chamomile, linden, and mint / regular tea.
• a shot glass of spirits or homebrew.

*Eating:*
• garlic / red beets.

*Applying:*
• soaking in a warm bath, with or without herbs (burdock or chamomile leaves) and then going to bed well covered with quilts.
• going to bed early and resting as long as possible.
• cups (dry or wet) or leeches to get rid of "bad" blood.

## *Menstruation*

Menstruation, defined by a woman's monthly period, showed her that she was capable of reproducing and that she was not pregnant. During the early days, discussion of this natural female process was typically not an acceptable topic in mixed company, and most men found it too embarrassing to hear about its details. In some families it was an avoided topic of discussion, even between mother and daughter, until the daughter got her first period. Even then, only the most basic information might be shared. Most women were taught that menstruation was their "curse" to bear in life, and any associated pain or discomfort was to be suffered without complaint or expected pity. A missed period was of major concern to a woman because it was the first evidence of pregnancy, which most often was unplanned.

Daily hard physical farm work meant that a woman's menstrual blood flowed easily and that clotting was not usually a problem. Blood clots were associated with considerable abdominal pain. Minor menstrual discomfort was tolerated silently, and did not impede a woman's work. Women who experienced very painful periods, with severe pelvic cramping or deep aching pains, sought different forms of relief. These included:

*Applying:*
- bed rest.
- a hot pack on the abdomen.
- heat from lying on (indoors), or in (outdoors), a **clay oven**.

*Drinking:*
- a shot glass of alcohol (brandy, whisky, or moonshine / homebrew) in a cup of hot water.
- 1 tbsp. wormwood infusion, in a shot glass of wine; could be safely taken 3-4 times a day.
- a half to full cup of hot water.
- *Drinks* made from **ginger** *(imbyr)* / **yarrow** / **chamomile** flowers / calendula flowers / plantain leaves / raspberry leaves / or wormwood tops.

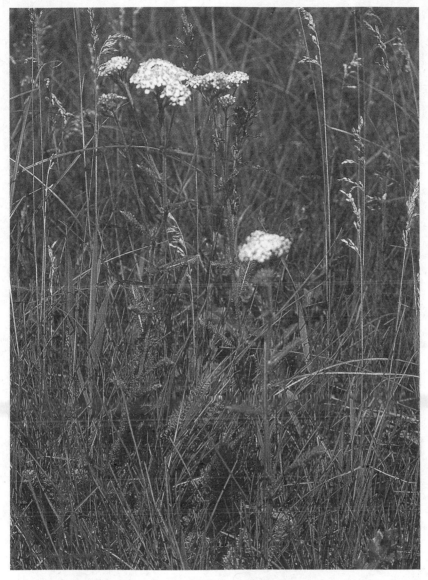

Yarrow poultices were used to stop bleeding and help wounds heal. [M. MUCZ]

- decoction of caraway seeds.
- concentrated raspberry juice for very painful cramps.

## Birth Control and Abortion

Most of my informants did not volunteer information or wish to discuss these topics. At best, these issues were referred to with indirect comments that were not elaborated upon because of their religiously sensitive nature. Even in current times, such topics are not openly discussed, least of all between men and women, so it is easy to understand the difficulties my elderly informants had in addressing these issues with me. Women, because of their willingness to share personal concerns and issues with other women, undoubtedly did discuss these matters with one another. Practical suggestions for both birth control and abortion were very likely shared with women in poor health, or those with large young families and limited resources.

The most natural form of birth control would have been one requiring the male to withdraw before ejaculating. This technique, which typically has a high failure rate, is still a widely used form of contraception in many rural areas of developing countries. Contraceptives, such as condoms, probably were not much used by the settlers because they would have been generally unavailable in rural areas, were costly, or might have been viewed as undermining a man's masculinity. Women often nursed their children until the age of three or four, and this practice was known to reduce the likelihood of conception. Large families and high pregnancy rates were evidence that contraception was generally not widely practised, or at best ineffective.

Abortion is an extreme form of birth control still widely used in many societies. If conception cannot be prevented, then this method ensures that the fetus does not develop to term. Herbal infusions or decoctions that would cause or promote menstrual flow, and the subsequent expulsion of the fetus, could have been used in the early stages of pregnancy when only the woman knew that she was pregnant. Available herbs, such as caraway, feverfew, ginger, lovage, juniper, parsley, rue, tansy, thyme, wormwood, and yarrow are known abortificants. Ergot, a fungus growing on rye, could also produce an abortion. Women would have been cautioned not to use these materials when pregnant and therefore would have realized their potential effect if used intentionally. Other herbs, preparations, or materials that could terminate a pregnancy would also have been secretively, but willingly, shared by those who understood a woman's desperation to not bear another unplanned child.

Abortion in later pregnancy could also have been induced, intentionally or accidentally, through hard work or heavy lifting. Such activity would have produced strained abdominal muscles and associated muscle spasms. Jumping off a fence or from a tree might also have caused enough of an internal shock to induce a spontaneous abortion. In extreme cases it is also likely that desperate women sought out more physical and internal intervention by someone in the area who knew how to do it. Such a practice would have been highly secretive and carried out with considerable risk to the pregnant woman. Local midwives, skilled in dealing with pregnancy and birthing, might also have been pressured into providing alternative services to women for whom another pregnancy was possibly life-threatening or highly unbearable under existing conditions. In any case, one must assume that these clandestine practices were not readily shared with others, but many women would have understood and accepted their necessity under the circumstances.

I vividly recall one informant describing, with both anger and tears, the painful memories of her poor mother seemingly constantly pregnant and the hardships it brought to her already-difficult life. The unkind comments she made about her father left no doubt that the pregnancies were not planned and certainly not of her mother's choosing. Large families were certainly a practical necessity of early homestead life, but they also exacted a toll, often a lethal one, on the women who bore the children.

## Pregnancy

Inadequate means of birth control, coupled with high infant mortality and the need for a large farm work force, resulted in a high pregnancy rate during the early settlement period. Children seemed to "arrive" on a regular basis, since most brides were both young and highly fertile. Contraception and family planning, as discussed previously, were not widely or successfully practised.

Pregnancy is stressful physically, emotionally, and physiologically. It is associated with an increase in appetite, breast enlargement, fatigue, the nausea of morning sickness, and irritability. Ongoing household and farm work demands meant that it was but another strain that a farm wife had to bear and suffer through. Like many other female health issues, it was also not openly discussed or described by my elderly informants. They undoubtedly viewed such suffering as a natural part of life but were not comfortable discussing it openly, especially with a man. To their credit, the women did deal with it quite successfully, but at a great personal price of stress and discomfort.

The seemingly more "delicate" health of women is often used as evidence for labelling them as the weaker sex. Some individuals even believed that having a daughter would result in a more difficult and exhausting pregnancy for the mother. Women therefore were inclined to hide, or at least minimize, the physical and emotional signs of pregnancy and attempted to carry on with their normal activities and workload. Regular pregnancies, coupled with hard physical work, were effective in keeping women at a disadvantage and in their "rightful place" in farming society. Multiple sequential childbirths not only deteriorated a woman's health during pregnancy, but also added considerably to her already heavy workload thereafter.

Children were often kept ignorant about the pregnancy, and its occurrence might be signalled only by the arrival of the midwife or doctor. Doctors, because of accessibility and cost factors, were rarely involved unless there were difficulties with the pregnancy or anticipated problems in the delivery. For most women, birth was seen as a natural event best carried out at home in a familiar setting. Home deliveries also allowed the woman to continue working until the last possible moment and to also resume work as soon as possible thereafter. A newborn was but a momentary joy, before the harsh reality of everyday life took over again and the baby became another task to manage.

Bloc settlements had at least one older woman who understood the features of pregnancy and birthing and was available to serve as a midwife. Years of dealing with her own pregnancies and deliveries provided invaluable experience in her being able to help others. Such wise elderly women knew what to expect, how to deal with it, and how to reduce the stresses of pregnancy and delivery. Younger women, especially first-time mothers, would often find it a painful and frightening ordeal. Their fears and concerns were further heightened if they did not have the comfort of a mother's, or older woman's, advice and support. Nevertheless, youth had its advantages: a healthier and stronger body dealt with the stresses of pregnancy and childbirth more easily.

A widely used tonic, taken daily during the latter stages of pregnancy, was any raspberry-based drink, which was believed to produce an easier and safer delivery. It was taken in the form of a raspberry-leaf infusion, a decoction of raspberry cane tips, or an equal-parts mixture of raspberry juice and hot water. Eating fresh or preserved raspberries was also considered effective.

> *When a woman was pregnant* (vahitna), *the older women told her to use raspberry* (malyna) *fruit tea every day. This was supposed to help her have a safe and easy birth* (narodzhennia). — J. K. / Vegreville

Morning sickness could be controlled by eating dry bread or salty foods such as pickles or sauerkraut. Food filled the stomach, reduced nausea, and provided essential minerals for both mother and fetus. The food's saltiness created a thirst that required greater fluid intake. Even drinking warm water helped a woman relax and stay hydrated. Nausea could also be reduced by using an infusion of mint leaves. Aches and pains in the lower back could be reduced with gentle massage or the application of hot, moist packs. Fatigue, common in the latter stages of pregnancy, could be reduced by drinking a cup of warm milk with an egg and a teaspoon of cinnamon beaten into it. Half a shot glass of alcohol before bedtime was believed to be a stress reliever that led to a better night's sleep.

Urinary difficulties were treated by placing onion peels into boiling water and squatting over the infusion's steam. The genitals were gently steamed in this manner until the urge to urinate was felt. The physical act of squatting may have been enough to create this urge and the steam merely provided additional relaxation.

## Childbirth

In the early homestead period, home births were the normal practice in rural areas. Doctors and hospitals were either not readily accessible or were too costly, so midwife-assisted home delivery was common. If a midwife was unavailable, an older female relative, a neighbour, or even the husband could provide the necessary assistance for an uncomplicated birth. More complicated pregnancies and deliveries required a doctor's intervention, but even then a midwife was

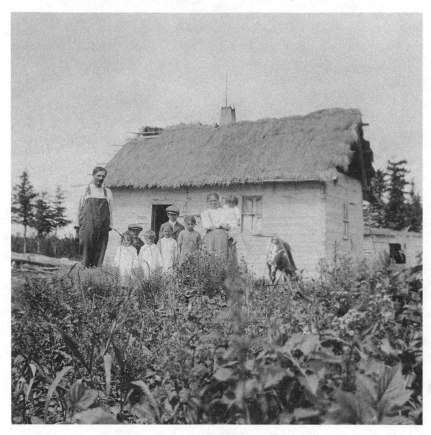

Children were a regular addition to a settler's family. [PAM N11632]

often sought out. Her experienced help was invaluable, and she also was able to learn additional skills from the doctor.

When a woman was near the end of her pregnancy, a local midwife would be sent for and would begin preparations for the home delivery. In winter, a bed would be placed in a corner of a room and a sheet hung around it to ensure privacy from peering young eyes. In summer the children would be sent out of the house until the delivery was over. It is not difficult to see why young children believed that their new sibling was brought by a stork or by the newly arrived midwife. Although delivery conditions in most homes were basic, the comfort of being in a familiar setting and surrounded by familiar faces more than offset most shortcomings.

Most home deliveries were routine procedures, and only premature births, prolonged labour, or unnatural positioning of the baby would have created any serious complications. Problematic deliveries, if unattended by a doctor, often resulted in the death of the infant and in many cases of the mother as well. Delivery complications, or health problems in the child's first year or two, resulted in high infant mortality rates in rural areas. In large families, it was not uncommon to have one third to one half of the children not survive to adulthood. Women also suffered greatly from the hazards of childbirth, and many men outlived two or three wives.

In a normal home delivery, if the water (amniotic fluid) had not "broken," the midwife might try to induce this by rupturing the sac with a wing feather. If sanitary procedures were not used, the mother could easily contract blood poisoning and die from this procedure. Extensive pain associated with prolonged or hard labour was often alleviated by having the mother drink a decoction of hemp seeds. If stronger contractions were required, these could be induced by having her drink a wormwood-seed tincture.

> My sister was pregnant (vahitna), and the hot summer weather, plus the baby's delayed birth, made her very sick. We called the midwife, and when she saw my sister's condition, she decided to "force" the birth. She went into the yard and found a chicken's wing feather, which she used to "break her water." My sister became very ill (slaba) after the delivery, and eventually died (pomerla) of blood poisoning. So you see what a midwife could also do. — S. T. / Vegreville

If the placenta was not expelled after delivery, a pail of oats could be placed on heated bricks and covered with hay. Water was poured over the hay and oats to create herbal steam, which the woman stood over. This induced expulsion of the placenta. Excessive uterine bleeding was controlled by drinking an infusion of nettles, but more serious internal hemorrhaging was treated by drinking a decoction of three-flowered avens roots, which was used for a week. In cases of severe post-delivery cramping, the woman was kept in bed and well covered with quilts and blankets. She might also be placed on (indoors) or in (outdoors) a clay baking oven. A chamomile infusion drink was often used to relax the mother and enhance breast milk production. In cases where her abdominal muscles were strained and weakened from the delivery, or because of numerous previous deliveries, a special treatment was used. An elderly female healer would be called in to massage the abdominal muscles back into place and use cloth strip bindings for support. This allowed the muscles to heal and recover their tone.

The newborn was often given two teaspoons, drop by drop with a tiny spoon or directly from a bottle, of **chamomile** or feverfew infusion. This was used to clean out its stomach before it received any milk. In some cases, the infusion was given for the first few days, prior to any breastfeeding, to tone up the baby's stomach for digestion. The dose could even be increased, to two to four tablespoons daily, if the baby was not feeding well or if the mother did not produce much breast milk. This infusion was also given if the baby had to be fed cow's milk, in cases where the mother died during childbirth or was not lactating adequately. The infusion might be the only nourishment available to the infant for a number of days if no cow's milk was available. Chamomile was believed to not only strengthen the digestive system, but also to make the baby grow healthier. If the mother developed mastitis, an inflammation of the breast tissue, this reduced lactation as well as her ability to breastfeed. This condition was treated by wrapping a warm or cold fresh cabbage leaf on the affected breast.

To help keep the infant's eyes clean during the first few days, the mother might squirt a bit of her breast milk into its eyes. To keep the baby clean, it was typically bathed in the morning and evening. After each bathing, sweet cream or unsalted butter was gently rubbed onto its body to protect the skin. Massage, as well as gentle manipulation of the arms and legs, was helpful in expelling any built-up gas and greatly reducing colic symptoms. In winter, the baby was kept warm by placing heated bricks, wrapped in towels, around its body.

A relatively easy delivery, typically possible for a young and healthy woman, meant that she could be up and about doing light housework, such as cooking, washing, and general cleaning, that same day or at least within a few days. It was not unheard of for her to be doing even heavier work, such as field work, gardening, or house plastering, in as little as a week or two after childbirth. The baby would be looked after by older siblings or, if necessary, brought out to the work site and kept sedated with poppy infusion (described in chapter nine). Once born, the infant was quickly assimilated into the household's routine.

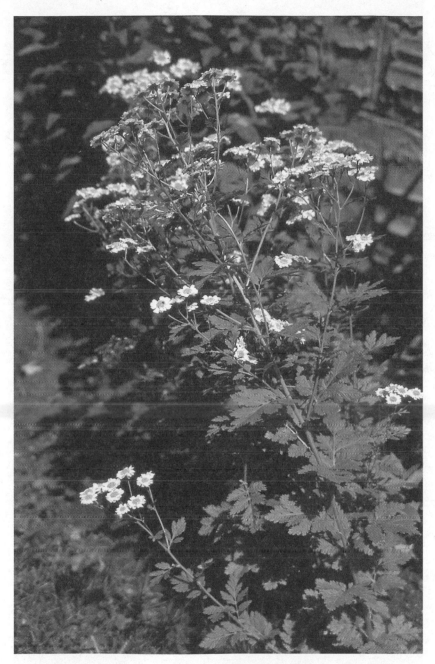

Chamomile was used in a wide variety of treatments. [M. MUCZ]

Although its basic needs were met, homestead life prevented the baby from being too pampered and fussed over, since it was now simply another "job" for someone in the household.

In unattended deliveries, the husband—who was more likely to be able to speak English—was often responsible for registering the birth. In many cases this was done at a much later date, due to unfavourable seasonal travel or work conditions, and many of these self-registered birth dates were inaccurate. At other times the birth was not registered until after the baby was christened, and sometimes the christening date was registered as the birth date.

## FEVER

A fever is the body's normal defensive response in dealing with microbial pathogens. It is usually a sign of an infection and often is a symptom of some serious illness. A rise in normal body temperature, accompanied by shivering, sweating, headaches, nausea, an upset stomach, and either constipation or diarrhea, are commonly associated with a fever.

Traditional Ukrainian healing often used the approach of inducing an even higher body temperature in order to "sweat out" the illness. This was typically done by covering the patient with numerous quilts and blankets or having them sit, fully clothed and in their outerwear, near a hot stove or oven. Food intake during this "sweating treatment" was greatly reduced, and intake of fluids, such as fruit juices or cold boiled water, was increased considerably to offset water lost through perspiration. In effect, this simple strategy both "heated and starved" the fever into submission, while maintaining body fluids at essential levels.

If the fever became dangerously high, was prolonged, or became impairing, it was often reduced by using such treatments as:

*Drinking:*
- *Infusion* of feverfew flowers / pineapple weed flowers / **chamomile** flowers or roots / sunflower tops / willow bark / parsley shoots (summer) or roots (winter) / mint leaves / caraway seeds / regular tea.
- *Fruit juice:* taken in concentrated (adult) or diluted (child) form, of highbush cranberry / **strawberry** *(sunytsi)* / raspberry / saskatoon berry /

blueberry. A few tsp. (child) or tbsp. (adult) of poppy infusion could be added as a pain sedative.
- *Decoction* of a few tbsp. wormwood in a cup of water (adult) / liquid from cooked and strained barley and oats (infant).
- *Milk*: warm / boiled with mashed garlic mixed in / warm with a mixture of honey, whisky, and baking soda / sour with ½ tsp. baking soda added.
- *Lemon juice* (or vinegar if lemons not available) mixed equally with cold or hot water / juice mixed with hot water and honey (child).
- *Vinegar:* ½–1 tsp. added to boiled water and ¼–½ tsp. baking soda— the solution consumed while it was still fizzing: 1 tsp. (child) or 1 tbsp. (adult).
- *Soup:* **chicken** / sauerkraut.

Throughout the day, all liquid drinks were taken in one- to three-cup doses, depending on the degree of dehydration suffered.

### Eating:
- 1 tbsp. sugar to which was added a few drops (more would cause vomiting) of kerosene.
- *Fruit*: cooked blueberry / strawberry / cranberry.
- cooked garlic / horseradish.

### Applying:

Infants and children:
- grated fresh potatoes to the feet, wrapped on with a moist cloth / crushed buckwheat *(hrechka)* moistened in cold water and wrapped on the feet / honey all over the body; the child was then wrapped in blankets and kept in bed.
- crushed garlic on the soles of the feet, rubbed in before covering the feet with woollen socks / whisky to the forehead, rubbed in / an equal mixture of water and vinegar to the forehead / a mixture of gunpowder (removed from shotgun shells) and goose fat rubbed on the body.
- grated potatoes or sliced onions placed in a moist cloth, wrapped on the forehead or wrapped around the chest and back / a cold wet

compress or cloth dipped in a healthy child's urine, wrapped (loosely or tightly) on the forehead.

- towel or flannel (non-itching) blanket dipped in very cold water, wrung out, and wrapped around the naked body. The cloth was changed when it warmed, and the treatment was repeated three times a day.

Adults:
- grease, which protects the skin, on the chest, arms, and soles. These areas were then rubbed with crushed garlic and wrapped in a warm blanket / whisky on the chest and feet and vinegar on the forehead, neck, soles, and palms / sauerkraut leaves or sliced potatoes (baraboli) around the forehead, wrapped on with a moist cloth. Leaves were replaced when warm, or revived by soaking in cold water; potatoes were replaced when they warmed or darkened.
- powdered mustard to the inside of woollen socks, which were then worn to bed.
- cups (wet or dry) to the arms, or leeches to the legs, to remove "bad" blood.

Depending on the availability of water, a child's body temperature could be lowered by gently washing the forehead and body with a cloth soaked in cold water. Adults could achieve the same result by immersing themselves in a tub of cold water.

## GASTROINTESTINAL PROBLEMS

Stomach and digestive problems were common due to poor food quality, storage, and preservation. Eating poorly preserved or spoiling foods, very rich or fibrous foods, questionably edible wild mushrooms, and excessive amounts of wild fruits, and drinking contaminated water would have contributed to some form of digestive upset. Less serious problems might have been caused by emotional distress or eating too quickly. Any of these developments would have led to abdominal pain, bloating, diarrhea, loss of appetite, and other digestive upsets.

Adults would have been capable of suffering the inconvenience, but children, especially the younger ones, would have been highly distressed by what was happening to them. Often a degree of relief could be achieved by induced vomiting (described later in this chapter) or by having the abdominal area gently massaged. A hot pack on the stomach would provide relief, but such treatment could prove dangerous if the source of the problem was really an inflamed appendix.

## Lack of Appetite

Physical work on a homestead or farm, coupled with plenty of fresh air, made the lack of an appetite an uncommon problem. People could not understand why a person would not want to eat, especially if they had been working hard. It was said that if you didn't eat today, then by tomorrow you would surely want to eat. A more common problem was not having enough to eat, let alone not having an appetite. Loss of appetite was therefore associated with a person's not feeling well or having some illness.

Various home remedies were used to strengthen and enhance the appetite and to settle the stomach, which helped digestion. These included:

### Drinking:
- a shot glass of alcohol (homebrew or wine), often taken by men before their main meal.
- 1 tsp. of wormwood infusion, in a glass of water, taken daily before each meal.
- ¼–½ cup pickle / sauerkraut / fermented or unfermented fruit juice.
- a cup of regular tea, with a pinch of black pepper / rose petal tea with honey.
- a shot glass of Watkins tonic.
- a glass of milk with a raw egg beaten in it.

### Eating:
- sliced or mashed garlic cloves, with vegetable oil, on bread or with the meal / grated horseradish as a side dish at a meal.
- raw onions on bread.
- boiled flax.
- fresh young dandelion leaves.

## Abdominal Upset

Stomach and intestinal upset was a common problem, as evidenced by the large number of remedies to treat the symptoms. Poor food sanitation and/or storage were the main causes of an upset digestive system. Such health conditions were usually short-term inconveniences and generally not life-threatening. Home remedies primarily involved drinking fluids, which helped alleviate the pain and resolved the source of upset. The treatments included:

*Drinking:*
- *Infusion* taken 3-4 times daily, of **chamomile** flowers (child) / strawberry leaves / **wormwood** tops (adult) / raspberry leaves or roots / buttercup flowers / mint leaves / yarrow tops / alfalfa flowers / centaury plant leaves / ginger root / lovage tops / marjoram tops / gentian tops / feverfew tops / burdock leaves or roots / turnip roots / pineapple weed flowers / chrysanthemum flowers / caraway seeds / anise seeds / corn silk / parsley leaves or roots / parsnip roots or tops / dock leaves (child) / Canada or sow thistle tops / Seneca root / thyme leaves / linden flowers / nettle leaves / senna leaves / rose petals / or regular tea. To any of these liquids could be added ¼-½ tsp. black pepper. A sweetener (sugar or **honey**) was often added to make the bitter drinks easier for a child to swallow.
- a shot glass, taken hourly, of a wormwood-leaf concentrate added to a cup of hot tea.
- *Fruit juice* taken in concentrated form, 2-3 times daily, in doses of a shot glass full (or 1 tsp. or 1 tbsp., if alcohol was added), of strawberry / blueberry / lowbush cranberry / raspberry / or chokecherry.
- *Sour drink*, taken in shot glass (child) or cup (adult) portions, of **pickle** *(marynovani ohirky)* or **sauerkraut** *(kysla kapusta)* juice / whey / or fresh cabbage juice. Raw eggs could be added to make the drink easier on the stomach.
- a cup of buttermilk or sour milk.
- *Alcohol:* a shot glass (adult) or 1-2 tbsp. (child) unadulterated homebrew / a shot glass (adult) of homebrew with 1 tbsp. pickling spice infusion / a shot glass (adult) of homebrew mixed with a ¼-½ tsp. black pepper /

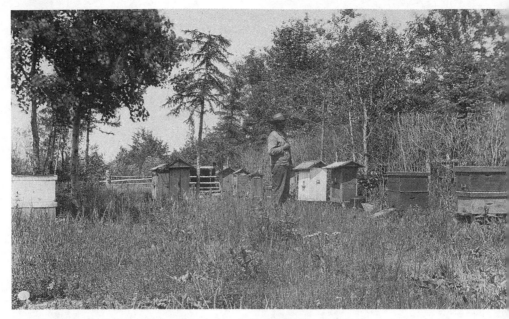
Honey was readily available and a common home remedy ingredient. [PAM N11590]

a bit of black pepper in 1–2 tbsp. homebrew (child) / 1 tbsp. of homebrew
in a glass of milk / 1 tsp. ginger powder in a shot glass of homebrew.

- *Tincture,* taken in doses of a shot glass each hour, made from wormwood
leaves / burdock roots / or chamomile flowers.
- *Milk:* a glass of warm or hot milk diluted (1:1) with water / with a raw
egg mixed in / or with 1 tsp. unsalted butter.
- *Fizzy drink* made from 1 tsp. baking soda mixed in a glass of boiled
water / 1 tbsp. vinegar, 1 tsp. sugar, and ½–1 tsp. baking soda in a glass
of water (drunk while it was still fizzing).
- a glass of water with 1 tsp. Epsom salts.
- *Decoction* of boiled flax seeds, taken in small quantities, over the day.
- *Hot drink:* a cup of strong coffee with ½ tsp. black pepper mixed in /
a cup of warm water / ¼ cup of warm water with ¼ tsp. black pepper /
a cup of hot water with 1 tsp. lemon juice and cream of tartar / a cup of
hot water with 1 tsp. Watkins or Rawleigh internal liniment.
- 1–2 tbsp. cod liver oil.

*Eating:*

- *Fruit,* fresh, dried, or rehydrated **blueberry** *(chornytsia)* / lowbush cranberry / raspberry / strawberry / or rhubarb; dried and boiled purchased fruits such as apples / prunes / or raisins.
- raw garlic, onions, or grated horseradish as a side dish with a meal.
- *Herbs:* chopped, fried, and scrambled with eggs: chrysanthemum leaves / chamomile flowers / mint leaves.
- a few drops of Watkins or Rawleigh internal liniment on 1 tbsp. sugar.
- boiled flax seeds in cereal or eaten raw and washed down with a cup of boiled water.
- sauerkraut / fresh cabbage cores / cooked parsnip roots.
- burnt bread.
- crushed juniper berries mixed with sugar. Used in doses of 1 tsp. for a young child and 1 tbsp. for an older child.
- 1 tsp. goose fat.

*I was not feeling well (dobre) and could eat nothing more than a piece of dry bread. Eating anything else made me feel bloated and sick. A man in our area knew a lot about wild plants and how to heal with them. My husband went to him and described my condition. He suggested trying wormwood (polyn) and gave my husband a paper cone full of roots (korinnia) and another cone of flowers (kvity), which were to be used in preparing a strong tea. The root portion was to be boiled for five minutes and then a portion of the flowers was to be added to the hot solution. I was to drink this bitter tea, three times a day, before each meal. It was very bitter, but it did work and I could soon eat without any further problems. — K. N. / Smoky Lake*

## FOOD POISONING

A lack of proper food storage facilities, especially in the summer, meant that eating spoiling or spoiled foods could easily cause severe stomach problems from food poisoning. Similarly, inadequate food preservation meant that food stored for long periods could go bad. If only mild food poisoning was suspected to be contributing to the digestive upset, then the person might settle their stomach by:

*Drinking:*

- small portions of pickle or sauerkraut juice.
- vinegar.
- Epsom salts solution.
- a few drops of kerosene on sugar.

## VOMITING

An upset stomach was typically relieved by natural or induced vomiting of the materials causing the upset. It was not uncommon for an innocent and adventurous child, or an inattentive adult, to ingest a hazardous household or farm product such as formaldehyde or gasoline. These chemicals were highly toxic, and immediate purging by either physical means or by swallowing something to induce vomiting was critical.

Treatments used to induce vomiting included:

*Drinking:*

- fresh milk / sour milk / or milk mixed with fine chicken, goose, or duck feathers.
- whites of four fresh eggs
- salt water solution.
- ½ tsp. dry mustard mixed in a cup of water.
- 1–2 tsp. kerosene.

The above drinks, taken a cup or more at a time, had to be consumed as quickly as possible.

*Applying:*

- two fingers to the back of the throat.
- large feathers down the throat.
- two arms, placed around the body and under the stomach, squeezed to create an upward motion.

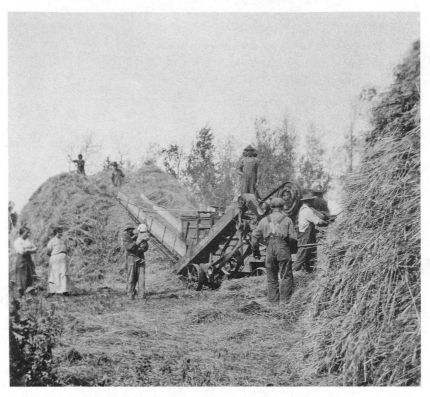

Threshing was dirty, hard, and dangerous work. [PAM N9241]

*One day my brother* (brat) *was walking home from school and became very thirsty. He noticed a jug sitting by the threshing machine, and he decided to take a drink from it. He quickly realized that it was gasoline and not water* (voda) *which he drank, but he did not mention this to anyone. He only said that he was not feeling well and wanted to go to bed. By suppertime he was coughing badly and we could smell the gasoline on his breath. The man running the threshing machine guessed as to what had happened but did not know what to do. My father, who was a well-read man, remembered an article* (stattia) *that said it was important to clean out the stomach when something like this happened. He had my mother make up a mixture* (mishanka) *of water and mustard, which my brother had to drink quickly. In a few minutes he ran out of the house and vomited everything out. What my father learned had worked.* — M. T. / Vegreville

Excessive vomiting associated with an illness was offset by drinking warm tea mixed with honey. This was done because it was important to drink as much liquid as possible in order to keep the body hydrated.

## Diarrhea

This condition produces frequent, abnormally soft and watery stools. The settlers called it a "running" stomach or simply "to go outside" *(ity nadvir)*. It is also associated with cramping and nausea, which indicate intestinal upset or possible digestive tract inflammation. For children this condition is more life-threatening because it causes a major loss of body fluids, salts, and nutrients. It was therefore taken more seriously and treated more aggressively in children, especially the very young. Adults would often let the problem take its course and suffer the inconvenience of frequent trips to the outhouse or bush.

Its treatments varied, but were similar to those for digestive problems. They included:

*Drinking:*
- *Infusion,* weak and sweetened with honey or sugar (child) or strong and plain (adult), made from **strawberry** roots or leaves / raspberry roots or leaves / wormwood tops / chamomile leaves and flowers / nettle leaves / mint leaves / cinnamon / ginger root / chamomile roots / parsley leaves / Seneca root / mixture of nettle and raspberry leaves / mint leaves and chamomile flowers. Regular tea, whose tannic acid content would tighten up the stomach and digestive tract, was also used. 1 tsp. dry tea, washed down with warm water, could be used in an emergency.
- *Juice:* concentrated and taken in tbsp. portions (sweetened with honey or sugar for children) from blueberries / chokecherries / strawberries / high- or lowbush cranberries / raw beets.
- *Liquid:* ½–1 cup strained fluid from boiled rice / pearl barley / rolled oats.
- *Water:* to make up for lost fluids: a cup of boiled water, with or without a half rennet tablet dissolved in it / a cup of water mixed with ¼ tsp. black pepper / a milky batter made from a mixture of flour and water.

- *Milk,* or its products, which help stiffen the contents of the bowel: a cup of **warm milk** *(teple moloko)* / sweet cream / a glass of milk with a beaten egg in it (child).
- *Alcohol:* a shot glass full with ½–1 tsp. black pepper (adult) / a few tbsp. of a homebrew and honey mixture (child).

*Eating:*
- *Fruit preserves,* with honey or sugar added for children, made from blueberries / high- or lowbush cranberries / any available dry berries and fruits / plantain fruit boiled in water.
- *Eggs:* hard **boiled** and **crushed** up, in portions of 1–2 eggs for children and 3–4 eggs for adults. An infant or very small child might be given boiled and mashed egg yolks, mixed (3:1) with potatoes.
- *Grain products:* dried bread soaked in milk (child) / boiled milk mixed with crackers and hard-boiled eggs (child) / a bowl of cooked rice / dried and burnt bread / crackers / bread sprinkled with 2 tsp. cinnamon.
- 1 tbsp. coffee beans, chewed slowly (adult).
- salted cottage cheese *(brynza).*
- mint oil on 1 tsp. sugar.

## HANGOVER

Widespread social use of alcohol, mainly spirits (whisky, homebrew) was rooted in Old Country traditions of hospitality and friendship. It was a common feature of home and community entertaining and often led to excessive consumption, especially by men. Its short-term effect on the body was a rise in blood-sugar levels, and its long-term effects were fat buildup in the liver and an overall wasting of the body. A major immediate consequence of its excessive use was a significant hangover the next day. This produced a throbbing headache, irritability, shakiness, fatigue, nausea, dizziness, and mild dehydration because of excessive urination or vomiting. Most individuals merely endured these side effects, for they were only temporary and disappeared in a few hours. Others for whom this was a relatively regular occurrence tried to find more immediate relief by vomiting or settling the stomach and head with various home remedies. These involved:

*Drinking:*

- chrysanthemum flower tea.
- strong coffee, which acted only as a diuretic.
- **pickle / sauerkraut** juice *(sik)*.
- salt water.
- 1-2 cups sour milk to induce vomiting / 1-2 cups fresh milk to settle the stomach.
- stale beer / half a shot glass of spirits to sedate the stomach.
- mouthful of urine, which was disgusting and quickly cleared the head.

*Eating:*

- plain sauerkraut / sauerkraut soup.
- salty pickles / pickled herring.
- brown bread.

*Applying:*

- fresh or fermented (sauerkraut) cabbage leaves on the forehead, bound on with a cloth.
- a cold, moist compress on the forehead.

## HEADACHE

Headaches were a common though relatively minor health problem. Daily tensions from running a household and farm, along with long exhaustive days working in the sun, brought on headaches. Dull steady pains around the head or extreme throbbing in the head or nasal areas were its indicators. More severe and prolonged migraine headaches also occurred. Lying down and resting would seem the simplest and most effective treatment, but a demanding work schedule prevented such possibilities. Unless onset occurred late in the day, a headache had to be endured or treated with home remedies. Only very severe headaches, such as migraines, were treated with complete rest in a darkened area, which proved to be the most effective remedy. Persistent headaches might be treated with supernatural healing.

*If someone in the family had a headache* (bil holovy), *Mother would get a cup of cold water and some charcoal from the wood stove. She would throw individual pieces of charcoal* (derevne vahillia), *while counting backwards from twelve, onto the water. The person with the headache would then be given some of this water to drink* (pyty), *and the rest of the water would be rubbed onto the head. It stopped the headache.* — N. S. / Viking

The wide range of home treatments included:

### Drinking:
- *Infusion* of mullein leaves and flowers / thyme leaves / red willow bark / linden flowers / **chamomile** flowers / caraway seeds / rosehips / nettle leaves / hemp leaves / mint leaves / hops / regular tea.
- a shot glass of spirits, preferably homebrew.
- a few tablespoons of wormwood concentrate, sweetened with **honey** or sugar, in a glass of water.
- juice of a chopped onion, mixed with a bit *(troshka)* of salt in 2 cups water. This was soaked overnight and then strained.
- 1 tbsp. Watkins or Rawleigh red liniment in ½ cup hot water.
- a few tbsp. concentrated raspberry or pin cherry juice, dissolved in a cup of hot or cold water.

### Eating:
- 2 tbsp. honey, eaten at each meal.
- a few cloves of garlic.
- 1 (child) to 2 (adult) drops of Hoffmann's Drops on a spoonful of sugar. This was used to prevent headaches or to reduce their severity.

### Applying:
- raw **potato** / beet / onion slices cut ¼-½ in. thick, dipped in cold water or vinegar and wrapped onto the forehead with a moist cloth. Slices were re-dipped, or changed, when they became warm or, for potatoes, when they darkened.

- grated, cool potatoes / beets as a poultice on the forehead. This was changed when it became warm; 2 slices of potato on each side of the forehead (on pressure points?) bound on tightly with a cloth.
- raw or fermented (sauerkraut) cabbage leaves in a moist cloth wrapped around the forehead. They were replaced, or re-dipped in cold water, when they warmed up.
- **concentrated** or dilute (1:1) vinegar onto the forehead or scalp.
- *Infusion,* into which a cloth was dipped, of rose petals / wormwood tops / chamomile flowers / lovage leaves / nettle leaves. The dipped cloth was then applied to the head.
- decoction of calamus root.
- sauerkraut juice / cold water, soaked into a cloth, applied to or wrapped onto the forehead.
- crushed garlic clove juice put on a cloth and wrapped on the forehead.
- *Leaves* of fresh Solomon's seal / nettle / coltsfoot, wrapped on the forehead.
- dry or moist cloth wrapped tightly around the forehead.
- used tea leaves in a moist cloth wrapped on the forehead.
- Watkins or Rawleigh ointment / vegetable oil, such as sunflower, rubbed onto the forehead.
- *Heated:* sand / grain / salt placed between layers of cloth and placed on the forehead.
- *Inhaling* the fragrance of freshly crushed chrysanthemum leaves.

These physical treatments were most often done in the evening, when it was also possible to lie down and rest in a darkened room or area.

*A man visiting my uncle said that he had a terrible headache and needed to get rid of it. He asked me to go into the house and got him a cup of vinegar* (otset). *He took it, poured it over his head* (holova), *and then rubbed it in well. His headache soon stopped* (nezabarom zupynyvsia). — P. K. / Two Hills

Migraine headaches were more serious problems and were treated by:

*Applying:*

- a number of cups (see section on bloodletting in chapter eight) on the forehead / 6-8 cups on the cheek and neck area. These removed the "bad" blood causing the migraine. The relief may well have been due to the reduction in blood pressure from the loss of blood.
- leeches, behind the ears, left on until they fell off when full of blood.


## KIDNEY AND BLADDER CONDITIONS

In the urinary system, the kidneys and bladder are major organs involved in ridding the body of toxins and maintaining its fluid balance. If kidney functioning became seriously weakened by disease and the problem became long-term, medical help was usually sought. If the problem was of a temporary nature, home remedies were tried.

The bladder, which stores urine, is vulnerable to infection. Women were more prone to such infections, but these were most often treated secretively and probably with some embarrassment.

A common symptom of kidney problems was lower back pain in the kidney area. Ukrainian settlers were extremely careful not to allow their lower backs to get chilled, and they attempted to drink plenty of liquids to maintain proper kidney functioning. The more preventative and curative home remedies to treat kidney and bladder problems were:

*Drinking:*

- *Infusion,* ½ cup taken 2-3 times daily, of **parsley** *(petrushka)* leaves and/or roots / corn silk / horsetail stalks / plantain leaves / parsley and wormwood leaf mixture / birch leaves / chamomile flowers / yarrow flowers / a combination of dried strawberry fruit mixed with chamomile flowers and rose petals.
- *Decoction,* ½ cup taken 2-3 times daily, of **parsley** roots / parsnip roots / asparagus stalks / turnip roots / black radishes / rosehips / juniper needles and berries. Concentrated wormwood was also used, in doses of 1-2 tbsp. (with a sweetener), first thing in the morning and last thing at night.

- a cup of cranberry fruit concentrate diluted in hot or cold water.
- *Juice* made from beets / parsnips / carrots.

Kidney stones were treated with a pine bud decoction made by boiling two teaspoons of pine buds in two cups of water. This was taken, half a cup at a time, after each meal.

A tincture of burdock roots was often taken, on a regular basis, as a preventative tonic.

> *People said that parsley (petrushka) was good for the kidneys (nyrky).*
> *My young granddaughter was suffering from a kidney problem, and anything*
> *the doctors tried did not work. Someone told my daughter (dochka) to boil up*
> *some parsley tea and have the child drink it every day. When she returned for*
> *a checkup, the doctor asked her what she was using to get so much better.*
> *She answered that it was not his medicine but the parsley that was helping her.*
> — P. K. / Vegreville

### Eating:
- beets / parsley / parsnips / garlic.
- chicken soup.
- *Fruit* of **cranberries** (fresh, boiled or preserved) / plums / prunes.

### Applying:
- a hot pack or cups (dry) to the lower back area.
- inhaling smoke from burning bearberry leaves.

Male urinary problems required taking a piece of straw and lubricating it by dipping it in soapy water. The straw was gently inserted into the penis's urinary tube (urethra) to allow the urine to flow out. Females with urinary problems crouched over the vapours of onion peels steamed in hot water. This position was maintained until the urge to urinate was felt.

Yeast infections in women were treated by washing the urogenital area with a yarrow infusion. This was done daily until the condition cleared up.

## LIVER AND GALLBLADDER CONDITIONS

Solutions to health problems associated with the liver *(pechinka)* and gall-bladder *(zhovchnyi mikhur)* were relatively unknown in the early days, even by the doctors. People developed yellowing of the skin and whites of the eyes (jaundice) and experienced severe abdominal pain from gallstones *(zhovchni kameni)*, but their origins were unknown at the time. If the condition persisted even after treatment with home remedies, then medical treatment was sought. The liver is a major organ, and serious problems in its functioning were often lethal.

The limited home remedies for the liver and gallbladder were therefore more preventative than curative. They included:

### Liver

*Drinking:*
- *Infusion* of mint leaves / strawberry roots / **wormwood** tops / gentian leaves / parsley shoots / rose petals / beet roots.
- juice of dandelion stems.
- a cup of a healthy person's urine.

Jaundice in infants was treated by giving the baby, for a few days, a few tablespoons of a tincture made from sparrow droppings (collected from beneath the thatched roof).

*Applying:*
- bathing in an infusion of wormwood.

### Gallbladder

*Drinking:*
- *Infusion* of horsetail stems / parsley leaves / wormwood tops.
- mixture (2:1) of olive oil and lemon juice.

- decoction made from 2 lb. horseradish, cut into 1-in. pieces, simmered for half an hour in a gallon of water, and strained. A cup of this liquid was consumed daily until the gallstone condition (pain?) cleared up. Half a cup was then taken daily, as a preventative against recurrence.

*Applying:*
- bathing in an infusion of mullein leaves.

## ORAL PROBLEMS

### *Sore Throat*

Sore throats were common in children, especially during cold weather, and were blamed on inadequate clothing and footwear. In some cases the sore throat was a more serious problem associated with inflamed tonsils (described in the following section).

Home remedies were used for any sore throat and were generally applied in the evening so the affected person might be able to get a restful night's sleep. The treatments were typically liquids, since eating irritated a sore throat.

Treatments included:

*Drinking:*
- a cup of hot milk with 1 tsp. or 1 tbsp. butter, lard, or **goose fat** plus honey and crushed garlic. Sometimes crumbled bread was added to make it more appealing to children.
- *Alcohol:* a shot glass of alcohol with 1 tsp. melted lard (swallowed quickly) / a shot glass (adult) or a few tbsp. (child) alcohol / a shot glass of equal parts honey and alcohol (swallowed slowly).
- *Infusion* of **chamomile** flowers / linden flowers / blueberry concentrate / Seneca root / ginger root / regular tea.
- *Water:* a cup of warm to **hot** *(hariacha)* water plain or with crushed garlic / 2-3 tbsp. red liniment / 1 tbsp. lemon juice or vinegar if no lemon juice available / a few tbsp. homebrew plus some honey and unsalted butter.

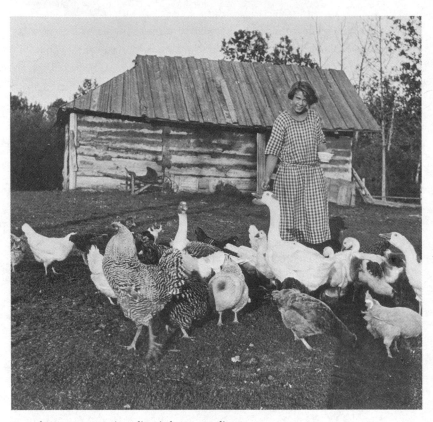

Goose fat was a common ingredient in home remedies. [PAM N5482]

- bowl of chicken soup.
- a cup of liquid, taken 1 tsp. at a time, strained from boiled flax seeds and mixed with a few tbsp. lemon juice and honey.
- 1 tbsp. warm honey.
- a cup of warm **milk** *(moloko)* or water with a few tbsp. of honey. The throat was then wrapped with a warm cloth or woollen sock.
- half a glass of strained liquid made by placing chopped onion into 2 cups salted water and soaking it overnight. This dosage was taken 3-4 times daily until the liquid was used up.
- a few drops of Watkins or Rawleigh red liniment or Hoffmann's Drops on 1 tbsp. sugar.

- 1 tbsp. red liniment in a cup of hot milk or **water** *(voda)*.
- concentrated cranberry juice diluted with water.

Liquids were consumed very slowly so that the surface of the throat would be well coated and warmed by them.

*Applying:*
- crushed garlic on the greased (goose fat or unsalted butter) neck and wrapping it with a woollen scarf, worn **sock** *(nosok)* or piece of flannel (non-itching) cloth or a warm, moist towel.
- medicated cream such as capsellina ointment, Watkins or Rawleigh red liniment.
- **goose fat**, lard, or extra-strength alcohol (homebrew).

The area was wrapped with a warm cloth, which was kept on overnight. This was done every night for a week.

- *Gargling* with a warm solution of **salt water** *(solona voda)* (¼–½ tsp. salt in half a glass of water) / chamomile flower tea or homebrew, which could then be swallowed for additional relief / kerosene in a glass of warm water with 1 tbsp. honey and 1 tbsp. vinegar / onion or garlic juice in warm water / an equal mixture of homebrew and vegetable oil in lemon juice, which could also be swallowed for added relief. This was typically done 3–4 times a day or every 2 hours.
- piece of pork fat, tied on a piece of string, swallowed and gently pulled back up. Repeated a few times., this coated the surface of the sore throat and reduced irritation.
- *Plaster* of **mustard** or grated horseradish placed over the greased neck.
- a hot pack (grain or salt) around the throat.
- steam to the head, which was breathed in slowly.

## Inflamed Tonsils

These presented a more serious problem and required surgical removal. A doctor visited schools annually and held a "tonsil clinic" for such a purpose. Tonsils, whether inflamed or not, were removed to prevent future problems, which could lead to the more serious rheumatic fever. Drinking hot liquids and keeping the throat warm was best way of reducing the pain of inflamed tonsils, but the only cure was removal.

Home remedies included:

*Drinking:*
- a cup of concentrated mullein-leaf tea.
- a cup of warm or **hot** milk containing 1 tbsp. unsalted butter or **goose fat**.
- a shot glass (adult) or a few tbsp. (child) of alcohol.
- warm or **hot** milk with 1–4 tsp. unsalted butter or **goose fat** plus crushed garlic.
- juice from 1 lemon added to a cup of warm or **hot** water.
- half a glass of pickle or sauerkraut juice.

*Eating:*
- 1 tbsp. crushed garlic mixed with a bit of cayenne pepper.
- pieces of raw garlic or onion. This was often crushed and placed on bread so children could more easily swallow it.

*Applying:*
- a hot pack on the throat.
- warm (woollen) cloth around the neck. A piece of pork fat could be placed under the cloth.
- the mouth of an open bottle of alcohol pressed against the throat, which allowed the alcohol to seep into the skin.
- gargling with salt solution (1 tbsp. salt to 1½ cups water), 3–4 times daily.
- garlic or onion oil infusion, placed over the back surface of the throat, with a wing feather.
- massaging the neck with red liniment or lard and then wrapping with a warm cloth.
- powdered sulphur to the back of the throat with a paper funnel.

*When I was eighteen, my tonsils became so swollen that talking and breathing was hard. Our neighbour* (susida) *came over to see what was wrong with me because she had not seen me around. When she saw my swollen tonsils, she said there was something that could be done for them. She went home and returned with half a bottle of whisky* (horivka). *I had to sit with a pillow behind my back, and place the neck of the open bottle tightly against the skin of my swollen throat, which allowed the alcohol to soak in. The area was soaked for a few minutes and then the bottle was switched to the other side of the neck. I did this for a full hour and ended up using half (equal to a quarter of a bottle) of the alcohol. When I woke up the next morning there was no swelling or problem with the tonsils because the alcohol had "burned" them out. A doctor later checked my tonsils and said that they were no longer a problem.* — M. K. / Smoky Lake

## Canker Sores and Inflamed Gums

These were treated by:

### Applying:
- honey.
- salt water.
- leeches.

## Dental Problems

Oral hygiene was poorly understood and seldom practised in the early settlement days. Sweets, such as sugar and honey, were not much available for general consumption but were commonly used to sweeten home remedies given to children. The sweet taste offset the bitterness of an ingredient and made the child more willing to take the medicine, especially since having a sweet treat was uncommon. Unfortunately, residue from sugary substances and other food collecting between the teeth often led to dental cavities, inflamed gums, swollen cheeks, and loose teeth. In the early days, dentists were unavailable in rural areas, and they also were seen as yet another expense settlers could ill afford. In emergencies, doctors extracted teeth.

Children often went to school in tears, struggling with the pain of aching teeth. The standard home treatment for such problems was to pull the teeth. The father would pull the children's teeth, since they were small and easily extracted. A bonesetter, or other local healer, provided a similar service for adults. Pliers or a piece of wire would be used on older children and adults, while a less-menacing string attached to the knob of an open door achieved the same result in younger children. The child was gently held by a parent, the door was quickly shut, and the problem tooth was thus removed.

> *A man came to my friend's place to pull out his grandfather's bad teeth. Before he started, he asked my friend to fetch a pail of cold water. The grandfather sat on a block of wood* (derevo) *and after his teeth had been pulled, the cold water* (zymna voda) *was poured over him. This was done to stop him fainting from the pain and the blood* (krov) *flowing from his mouth.* — F. H. / Vegreville

In some settlement districts, city dentists made regular three- to four-day visits to the area, and word quickly spread of their available services. In time, larger rural towns had permanent dental practices established, schools educated students about the value of good oral hygiene, and people had more resources to practise better dental maintenance and afford dental care.

> *An Indian once told me that to have healthy teeth* (zuby), *you had to chew on wood from a poplar tree that you saw being hit, and split open, by lightning* (blyskavka). *I actually saw this happen to a tree and took some of the wood splinters home for such use. Over the years, every month or so, I cut off* (vidrizav) *some small pieces and chewed on them for a couple of hours. I am ninety-one years old, have never had a toothache, and still have all my teeth except for a broken one.* — J. P. / Two Hills

Household treatments for painful teeth that were not immediately removed were relatively simple. Most often they consisted of applying an ingredient that acted as a sedative to the painful area. Home remedies included:

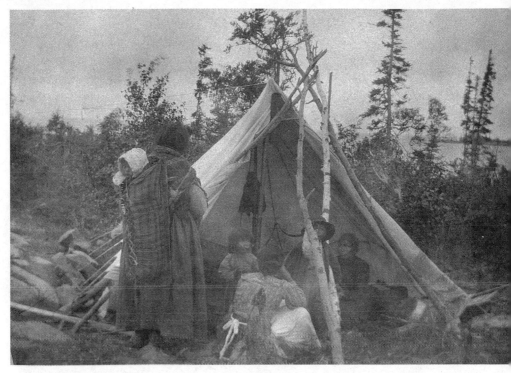

Aboriginal people travelled traditional trails and often camped on homesteads. [PAM N11579]

*Applying:*

- pinch of **tobacco** *(tiutiun)* / snuff / or chewing tobacco / a piece of unripe poppy head / a piece of cotton, soaked in poppy seed or resin tincture / ginger or cinnamon powder / whole or crushed cloves or their oil on a piece of cotton / salt, black pepper, or an equal mixture of salt and black pepper / cotton dipped into a tincture of black mullein seed or calamus root / a small wad of cotton, soaked in an infusion of oak bark or nettle tops / cotton, soaked in medicated ointment (capsellina?) / a boiled egg yolk / a piece of cotton soaked in kerosene or diluted carbolic acid / a piece of mint leaf, plantain leaf, or black henbane blossoms / salt water / tarry remains from brown burnt paper or scraped out residues from a well-smoked pipe / vinegar / a whole or crushed piece of garlic / a slice of raw onion / grated horseradish /

cotton dipped in homebrew (child) or holding a cheekful of homebrew (adult) on the area. Swallowing the excess undoubtedly assisted in reducing the pain.

- *Biting:* a piece of blue stone (copper sulphate) or crushed heated blue stone packed into the cavity / a moist cloth with salt and black pepper, which was bitten on to slowly release its contents.
- *Placing:* hot pack of **grain** *(zerno)* or salt on sore cheek for 10-15 minutes / fresh cow manure, in a moist cloth, wrapped onto swollen cheek / a piece of pork fat on the side of the cheek opposite to the side with the ache / Watkins or Rawleigh red liniment on a cloth.
- leech on the inflamed gum. Removal of blood from the area reduced the swelling and pain.
- steam, which was inhaled onto the tooth.
- *Smoke:* from burning black henbane foliage was allowed to flow over the painful area / holding a cheekful of cigarette smoke over the area.
- piece of garlic on the wrist, on the opposite side of the ache.


*My sister* (sestra) *became sick from infected teeth and developed a very swollen face* (lytse) *and a bad fever. The doctor was not able to do anything for her, and she went home to suffer with it. A visitor noticed her condition and suggested an unpleasant treatment. We had to collect fresh cow manure* (hnii vid korovy), *wrap it in a moist cloth, and then wrap it on her swollen cheek. We did this and regularly changed the poultice. In a few days my sister was well again.*
— S. S. / Camrose


## OUTDOOR HAZARDS

Insect bites, sunburn, and various skin rashes were hazards of working or playing outdoors, especially during the summer. Pests such as bees, wasps, hornets, horse-flies, and mosquitoes, which were known as "agents from hell," were a common problem for both humans and animals. Insect bites were more of a nuisance than a health hazard, unless the bite became infected from excessive scratching. Treatments were most often used for children or for sensitive individuals.

Otherwise, the bites were simply ignored. Summer's long, hot days also brought a risk of sunburn. Although hats or kerchiefs, long-sleeved shirts, pants, and long skirts were common field wear, exposed areas on the neck or hands could be burned.

Home remedies varied for different problems and included:

## Insect Bites and Stings

The most common treatment was to apply a knife blade or any other cold metal (a coin) to the bite and use it to scrape out the stinger. A bit of moist clay or soil also provided relief. The sting or bite, if it was irritating and itching, could also be rubbed with raw onion juice / baking soda paste / vinegar / or aloe vera sap. If nothing else was available, applying cold water provided some relief.

Bites that became infected or swollen due to an allergic reaction were treated with a poultice of plantain leaves or feverfew leaves. Bedtime relief, especially for children, was achieved by rubbing the affected areas with unsalted butter or cream.

## Sunburn and Heat Rash

A thin paste of blue clay, powdered and saved for such use, provided instant relief to sunburned areas. Similar treatment with cream or unsalted butter, which was more readily available, helped keep the skin moist and soft. Ointments, such as Watkins or Rawleigh products, or Vaseline, also provided relief. It was important to keep the burned skin moist and soft, which prevented cracking and blistering and possible infection.

> If a child (dytyna) had diaper rash or if someone developed a heat rash on
> the neck or in the groin area, then clay (hlyna) was used. Some blue clay was
> dug up, just above the water level, and this was smeared onto the skin (shkira).
> It brought instant relief, and if left on overnight, it helped the skin heal.
> — M. D. / Vegreville

## PAIN AND SUFFERING

Pain is the brain's method of alerting a person to the fact that some part of their body is not functioning properly or that it has sustained an injury. Its purpose is to reduce further damage, and its intensity and duration varies greatly. It may be minor and temporary, as that of an insect sting, or major and prolonged, as that of a severe burn. Pain sensitivity and tolerance also varies, typically being lower in children and greater in adults. A preoccupied person is also capable of increasing their pain tolerance and becomes less aware of pain over time. The early settlers' exhausting and diverse daily work schedules, coupled with a lack of pain-reducing medications, meant that in most cases they had to suffer *(terpity)* with and through their pain. Many times I heard this word *terpity* used when I asked what the last recourse was when all possible home treatments failed to reduce pain levels. As I listened to my informants use this term, I could feel its power and influence. It connected them to and made them aware of their body's condition, no matter how difficult it was to bear. Our modern society has become disconnected from pain, through the availability and use of a variety of pain relief medications, and we may be worse off for it.

Rest is generally sufficient for the body to recover naturally, but chronic pain requires attention. External muscle and joint pain was typically treated with hot packs or by soaking in hot baths. Home remedies for deeper internal pain were limited and, at best, could produce only a sedative effect. Remedies included:

### Drinking:
- *Infusion,* taken 3 times daily, of **chamomile** flowers / rosehips / feverfew / or peppermint.
- a few tsp. (child) or tbsp. (adult) of **poppy** tincture.
- a shot glass (adult) or 1 tsp./tbsp. (child) of alcohol.
- *Decoction:* a shot glass of **willow** *(verba)* bark (inner layer) / aconite roots / hemp seeds.

### Eating:
- unripe poppy seeds.

## PARASITES

Unsanitary and crowded living conditions, poorly preserved and undercooked foods, and limited personal hygiene were major factors in the occurrence and spread of parasites, both internal (pinworms and tapeworms) and external (head lice, body lice, bed bugs, and mites). Young children were especially vulnerable because of their tendency to play everywhere and with anything, put objects in their mouths, and pay little attention to personal cleanliness. Close personal contact during school and play, plus siblings' sharing clothing, meant that these infections spread quickly and widely. It was therefore a continuous battle to deal with such non-life-threatening but annoying health problems, as described below.

### Intestinal Worms

Pinworms are microscopic, round, worm-like parasites that live in the intestine and lay eggs around the anus. These were the most common internal parasite and spread easily among children. They were more of an irritant than a health hazard, and created no major health problems other than anal itching, which caused children to scratch and thus pick up the microscopic eggs on their finger tips. They then would re-infect themselves, or infect others, by contaminating any objects or food items they handled. Eggs could also be transferred to clothing or bedding and be passed on to others. With the exception of anal discomfort and itchiness, there are no outward symptoms of pinworm infestation. Good hygiene and keeping clothing clean are the best methods of controlling the problem and minimizing infection.

Tapeworms were less common but presented a more serious health problem. These macroscopic, long, flat, segmented worm-like parasites live in the intestines. They are usually aquired by eating improperly cooked meat (pork, beef, or fish) containing their cysts (larvae). Human infestation, in healthy individuals, typically causes few to no major symptoms. In young, elderly, or weakened individuals, symptoms such as abdominal pain, changes in appetite, diarrhea, and a pale complexion may develop. Passage of eggs through human waste contamination allows the parasite to spread to other animals and complete its life cycle.

*A child with tapeworms* (hlysty) *would become sickly, would not eat, and developed a pale complexion. This condition was treated by having the child sit on a "night pot" containing warm milk* (teple moloko). *It would sit on the pot until the tapeworms came out. You would not believe it, but you could see the worms in the pot and the child would soon feel better.* — M. P. / Edmonton

Various home remedies were used to treat parasitic intestinal worms, but most of the treatments used were for tapeworms. The various remedies were taken, three to four times a day, for a few consecutive days. These included:

**Drinking:**
- *Infusion* of chamomile flowers / tansy flowers / **wormwood** tops in doses of 1 tsp. in some milk (infant), 1-2 tbsp., with honey, in a glass of milk (child) or a few tbsp. or a shot glass (adult).
- a few tbsp. (child) or a shot glass (adult) of alcohol or wormwood tincture.
- a cup of sour milk or whey (child).
- ½-1 cup Epsom salts solution (adult).
- a few drops to 1 tbsp., proportioned to age, of kerosene on sugar or in water (child) / 1-2 tbsp. kerosene diluted (1:1) with water (adult) / 1-2 tbsp. syrup made from boiling equal portions of vinegar, sugar, corn syrup, and kerosene.
- 1 tbsp. Watkins or Rawleigh internal liniment or mint oil, taken with sugar (child) or water (adult).
- pickle or sauerkraut juice. This was given to a child, on an empty stomach, first thing in the morning.
- ½ cup syrupy beet decoction.
- concentrated fruit juices.
- 1 tsp. hemp seed oil.
- a cup of milk in which celery seeds had been boiled.

*One of my children had worms, and I gave her a teaspoon of kerosene* (has) *so that they would come out. The next morning she was crying* (plakala), *and*

*I could see a worm sticking out of her anus. I asked my husband to pull it out, and two long worms came out.* — M. M. / Edmonton

**Eating:**
- sour food such as **pickles** or sauerkraut.
- cinnamon powder spread on toasted bread or mixed into a pudding.
- lots of raw garlic or horseradish.
- ground tansy flowers mixed in food.
- dry fruits.
- 1 tsp. crushed juniper berries mixed with sugar.
- Sen-Sen (purchased from a general store or drugstore).
- powdered sulphur mixed into food or taken with a sweetener (sugar or honey).

*Our young daughter never told us that she was bothered by worms, and there was no way we could tell, either. One day when we had company, I opened a large jar of pickles* (marynovani ohirky) *and left them on the table. As the kids played they also ate them, but my daughter seemed to be eating quite a few. The next day as I was emptying out the night pot that she had used, I noticed two large worms* (velyki hlysty). *It is amazing how the body seems to "know" what it needs to rid itself of worms.* — J. K. / Innisfree

## Lice

### HEAD LICE

These are extremely small, wingless, flat insects that primarily infest the scalp. They are common on children and spread easily and quickly through personal contact or shared headwear and combs. The adult louse sucks blood from the scalp and leaves behind extremely itchy red spots, which can become bloody when scratched. Although adults live for only a few weeks, the female lays a few eggs (nits) daily on hair shafts and maintains the infestation.

*A ten-year-old boy had such an infestation of hair lice* (volosiani vushi) *that his head was bleeding. His poor mother was concerned that they might get into his eyes and cause more problems. She sent him to a neighbour to get a fine comb that was used to comb out head lice. She soaked his head* (holova) *in water and then carefully combed his hair. The lice were so thick that you could see them floating on the top of the water in the basin.* — A. B. / Camrose

Visits by children from an infested household, or more often through contact at school, meant that most children had to deal with head lice at one time or another. Outbreaks were usually first detected in the schools, where teachers were always on the lookout for any signs of aggressive head scratching or bloody scalps. In cases where there was a high incidence, or a recurrence, of a head lice infestation, remedial action meant thorough hair washing and very short haircuts. Teachers would commonly send a note home explaining what had to be done to eliminate the problem and would suggest the purchase of a special comb. These combs had very closely spaced teeth, which were capable of combing out the adult lice. It was also necessary to have all bedding, clothing, and headwear washed and kept clean. Children who were continually being re-infected, most likely from younger siblings, would be sent home from school until their condition cleared up. Such measures were necessary to ensure that the problem did not persist in the school.

Home treatments consisted of:

- *Combing out* the lice, with a specially purchased fine-tooth comb. The person's head was placed over paper, or onto a white apron on a mother's lap, and the adult lice carefully combed out. These were then killed by squashing them between the fingers.
- *Cutting* the hair extremely close to the scalp. Such a "pig shave" was typically done in the early spring when infestations were more common.
- *Washing* the hair in an appropriate solution and then combing it out. This involved soaking, for a ½-1 hour in the solution, rinsing off the solution with clean or **soapy** *(z mylom)* water, and then combing out the dead adult lice. Since the treatment did not kill the nits, it had to be repeated 1-3 times a week or even possibly every 5-6 days until the problem cleared

up. The wash solutions consisted of undiluted **kerosene** applied directly to the head or applied to a wet cloth and then rubbed on / a diluted (¼–½ cup in a pail or 1–2 tbsp. in a basin of water) kerosene solution / a diluted (a concentrated one could burn the skin and result in hair loss) infusion of stove ashes / a pure or diluted (¼ cup in a basin of water) solution of vinegar / wormwood infusion / strong homemade laundry soap.

*My daughter picked up head lice at school, and I treated her hair with a kerosene wash. I put in a bit of kerosene* (has), *enough so that I could smell it, into the wash water and left her hair soaked with it for a half to full hour. I then rinsed out the kerosene with clean water. The lice and eggs* (iaitsi) *would swell and burst from the treatment. Only one kerosene treatment was needed to get rid of the lice.*
— A. W. / Daysland

### BODY LICE

These are also very small wingless insects that feed on blood. Their bites leave small red areas that become very itchy and, when scratched, easily infected. They live and lay eggs on clothing but are not as easily spread as are head lice. Ukrainian settlers, relying on Old Country knowledge, believed that dogs were the sources of infestation, since dogs were always scratching themselves. Infestations were most common when people lived in overcrowded conditions, shared bedding, or had poor hygienic practices.

The most effective control method was to boil all infested clothing and bedding. Older children were made to drink, before each meal, a mixture of one teaspoon of wormwood infusion in a quarter cup of water. Young children would have fresh wormwood leaves wrapped on their abdomens and the herb's strong fragrance helped reduce the incidence of bites and let the children sleep better.

## Bedbugs

These larger, flat, wingless insects lived in crevices, or under wood bark on the posts of bed frames or log walls. They came out at night and sucked blood from sleeping bodies. They were generally spread by infested visitors who came to spend the night, or by infested visiting children playing on beds. They were a terrible problem *(bula bida)* once they became established in the house. They were extremely unbearable to young children, because their soft skin was an ideal feeding site.

The treatment to control and get rid of them involved washing all the bedding and pouring boiling water into all household crevices where the bedbugs could find shelter. Fumigating the house, with all of the doors and windows closed, was done by burning sulphur in a pail. Children were also rubbed down with fresh wormwood leaves—the oily residue would keep the bedbugs away for a time.

## Mites

These are small, eight-legged non-insect organisms with piercing and sucking mouthparts. They burrow under the skin to lay eggs, and these sites become intensely itchy and reddened. The resulting skin infection is termed scabies. Although their outbreaks were uncommon, they were easily spread through body contact or sharing of infested clothing or bedding. In school settings, their outbreak was termed the Seven Year Itch or the School Itch.

Treatment involved soaking the affected skin in water and then applying an equal mixture of lard and powdered sulphur / powdered sulphur and powdered blue stone (copper sulphate) mixed in lard. Regular treatment with either mixture cleared up the condition in a few weeks.

### RESPIRATORY PROBLEMS

Laboured or heavy breathing *(iadukha)*, which was uncommon, was associated with certain seasons (spring, fall) or environmental conditions (dust). Asthma and allergies, which both have this symptom, were poorly understood at the time. Excessively dirty, dusty, or smoky working conditions could cause lung inflammation and congestion in sensitive individuals and create breathing difficulties. Some believed this was also due to a reaction to certain foods, such as cow's milk. Progressive chest congestion, associated with the flu or a cold, could also produce short-term breathing problems.

More severe cases of breathing difficulties were taken to a doctor for medical attention, but home-based remedies were also used. These included:

### Drinking:

- *Infusion* of **wormwood** tops (sweetened with honey for children) / lobelia flowers / parsley leaves / young dill tops / a combination of dill and parsley / crushed oats / cayenne pepper / lily of the valley flowers / regular hot tea.
- a cup of warm milk with 2 tbsp. melted goose fat.
- a cup of goat's milk.
- a shot glass (adult) or 1 tbsp. (child) alcohol.
- 1 tsp. **kerosene** *(has)* or turpentine, placed on the tongue for slower absorption.

### Eating:

- fresh lily of the valley flowers.
- a few garlic cloves.

### Applying:

- steam to the **face** *(lytse)* or full body, generally with no herbs added.
- cuts to a vein to remove "bad" blood.
- cups (dry) to the chest area.
- alcohol on the chest, rubbed in.
- a hot pack or hot moist compress to the chest.
- Watkins or Rawleigh camphorated ointment, on a piece of cotton, into the nostrils.

## Congestion

#### CHEST

This was a common health problem during the winter and was often a sign of a developing cold or flu. It resulted in a hoarse cough because of bronchial irritation. Adults simply tolerated this irritating problem, but the condition was of greater concern in young children because it could lead to a more serious infection such as bronchitis or pneumonia.

Chest congestion was usually not treated as a separate problem, but as part of the overall treatment for a cold or flu. Most remedies involved a combination of both external and internal treatments, with liquid ingredients being most used. The treatment was generally applied at night, when the person could rest and be kept warm with quilts and blankets.

Home remedies varied, depending upon the type of condition being treated, and included:

*Drinking:*
- a cup of hot milk (child) or water (adult), with 1 tsp. badger *(borsuk)* or bear *(medvid)* fat in it.
- a cup of hot milk or tea with 1 tbsp. melted goose fat or unsalted butter mixed in and, for children, sweetened with 1 tsp. honey.
- a cup of hot water with 1 tsp. dissolved goose fat / or goose fat on a spoon, washed down with hot water / 1 tsp. or 1 tbsp. mashed garlic with the juice of a lemon added.
- a cup of hot milk or water with 1–2 cloves of crushed garlic in it.
- a cup of hot milk, water, or tea, with ¼–1 tsp. red liniment (patent medicine), sweetened with honey for children.
- a cup of hot water or tea with 1–2 tbsp. honey / mixed with 1 tbsp. butter and honey. 1 tbsp. lemon juice (child) or a shot glass of spirits (adult) could be added / a cup of hot lemon drink made from the juice of 1 lemon and topped off with hot water.
- a shot glass of homebrew and 1 tbsp. black pepper, in ¼ cup tea.
- *Infusion* of lily of the valley flowers / mint leaves / mullein leaves / nettle leaves and flowers (summer) or roots (winter) / raspberry leaves / **chamomile** flowers / feverfew leaves / linden flowers / **rosehips** or petals / Canada thistle flowers / red clover flowers / or thyme leaves.
- *Decoction* of birch leaves / crushed oats / ginger root / or raspberry canes (entire cane or only the inner bark).
- *Tincture* of unripe poppy seeds or pods / or chamomile roots.
- *Cough syrup,* taken in a 1 tsp. or 1 tbsp. dose, directly or in a cup of hot water. These were made from the strained liquids of concentrated birch sap (5–10 per cent of original volume) / sliced or chopped onions

covered with ½ cup honey or sugar, and left to sit overnight at room temperature / an onion decoction with sugar added to make it syrupy / a hollowed-out beet stuffed with sugar and baked until its contents liquefied / or a flax decoction with honey and lemon juice
- homebrew was used to induce sweating, taken unadulterated in doses of a shot glass (adult) or 1 tbsp. (child) / or mixed with mashed garlic and taken a shot glass at a time (adult), repeated 3 times daily / warmed beer.
- a few tbsp. (child) or ½ cup (adult) pure vinegar.
- a few drops of kerosene on 1 tsp. sugar.
- berry juice—**cranberry** preferred, made from dry berries in winter.
- chicken soup or broth.

Infusions, decoctions, tinctures, and homebrew remedies were taken three times daily, and the more bitter non-alcoholic ingredients were sweetened with honey for children.

### Eating:
- sliced or mashed garlic cloves on bread smeared with bacon fat and salted (adult) or unsalted butter (child).
- chopped onions heated in oil.
- cooked and ground beets mixed with garlic and a bit of sulphur.
- scraped horseradish, preserved in vinegar.
- mixture of crushed garlic, chopped onions, and honey cooked together, taken in tbsp. portions.
- 1 tbsp. honey.
- cough candy made from brown sugar, mixed with vinegar and butter, and then rolled into "pills" (child).
- a few drops of turpentine, or kerosene, on sugar (adult).
- a few Hoffmann's Drops on sugar.

### Applying:
- moist hot packs or compresses made from chopped onions fried in butter or lard. These were placed onto a flannel cloth and wrapped around a baby or infant's front and back.
- **mustard** or horseradish plaster.

- *Poultice* of hot flax seeds / crushed garlic / grated onion or raw potato; cups (wet) or leeches were used on adults and the elderly.
- *Rubbing* the body with crushed garlic and then covering it with a flannel cloth / **goose** or chicken fat applied to the skin directly, or first put on brown paper and then wrapped on with a cloth / bear grease / crushed garlic on the soles and goose fat on the chest and back / external liniment or ointment (capsellina?) / an initial layer of **goose fat**, lard or pork fat and then kerosene rubbed in / a mixture of kerosene and some type of fat / pure kerosene applied to the chest, throat, and beneath the mouth and nose / unsalted butter / or rubbing alcohol.
- soaking in a tub of hot water. This produced excessive sweating, which was maintained by consuming a shot glass of homebrew and being well covered in bed.
- *Inhaling* smoke from dried coltsfoot leaves burned on live coals / steam from heated water with an infusion of nettle leaves or a few tsp. red liniment.

External body remedies were most often applied to the chest, back, and soles of the feet. If garlic was used it could be irritating, so the skin was covered with some type of grease as a protective barrier.

### NASAL

Nasal mucous accumulation causes a stuffed up and runny nose that makes breathing and hearing difficult. This often clears up on its own in three to four days, but becomes quite irritating if it persists. A common home treatment was to keep warm by sitting fully clothed near a hot stove or going to bed well covered with blankets and quilts.

Other home remedies that were used included:

*Drinking:*
- mixture of equal portions of honey, lemon juice, and spirits in regular tea.
- 1 tbsp. at a time of honey and lemon juice added to the water strained from boiled flax seeds.
- a shot glass of alcohol in a cup of hot water.
- a shot glass of a mixture of alcohol and honey.
- 1 tbsp. honey and 1 tbsp. goose fat in a cup of hot milk.

- 1 tsp. at a time of a mixture of equal parts garlic and onion juice.
- **hot milk**, with mashed garlic and 1 tsp. butter or goose fat.
- 2 tbsp. raspberry or pin cherry fruit concentrate in a cup of **hot** or cold water.
- a cup of chicken broth.

### Eating:
- 1 tsp. melted goose fat.
- a few Hoffmann's Drops on 1 tbsp. sugar.
- horseradish / garlic / onion.
- a few tsp. of a cayenne pepper and honey mixture.

### Applying:
- a warm, moist cloth to the forehead and lying down.
- a hot, moist compress on the nose.
- a mustard plaster on the chest.
- rubbing either Watkins or Rawleigh camphorated ointment on the chest and under the nose.
- crushed garlic in a cloth sachet tied under the nose overnight.
- an old woollen sock over the nose.
- a few drops of camphor oil into the nose.
- steam to the head, for at least 5 minutes, from hot water containing: mashed garlic / camphor / Watkins or Rawleigh ointment / salt / mint / chamomile / hay screenings / spruce branches.
- hot water soak to the feet, and then wrapping them in a blanket.
- *Inhaling* snuff, which induces sneezing / fumes from mashed horseradish root or onions heating on the stove / smoke from hairs from the tip of a cat's tail or smoke from goose, chicken, or duck feathers placed on hot coals.

## Bronchitis

This is a viral or bacterial inflammation of the major air tubes (bronchi) in the lungs. It results in a narrowing of the air passages and produces a harsh cough that brings up yellowish green phlegm or sputum. Such an infection could be acute (short term) or chronic (long term). It was typically treated with:

*Drinking:*
- a heated mixture of crushed garlic, 1 tbsp. lard, and a shot glass of alcohol, 2-3 times daily.

*Eating:*
- grated horseradish root to heat up the chest.

*Applying:*
- steam, from a decoction of spruce or pine buds, directed to the head.

## Whooping Cough

This acute, contagious disease generally affects children. It develops from a bacterial infection of the mucous membranes lining the air passages of the lungs. Its onset is associated with a loss of appetite, a mild fever, and coughing. When fully developed it causes severe bouts of rapid coughing followed by an involuntary intake of air, which makes the distinctive "whooping" sound. The coughing can become so severe that it produces nasal or oral bleeding. The major symptoms lessen after one to two weeks, but the associated coughing can linger for an additional three to five weeks.

Its basic treatment was steaming, using a pot of hot or boiling water, the immediate area around the patient. This provided a degree of immediate relief for the chest congestion. The patient was also given a daily dose, for as long as the coughing persisted, of any of the following: a few drops of kerosene on a teaspoon of sugar, a teaspoon of badger fat washed down with hot milk, a cup of boiled milk with crushed garlic added, or mint-leaf tea with honey.

*My father had killed a badger (borsuk), which we used for food, but Mother also saved its fat for treating coughs and colds. A young neighbour of ours had whooping cough that was so bad it lasted throughout the winter (zyma). Since there was no doctor in our area, the girl tried different home treatments, but none worked. When my mother realized that girl's condition was not getting better, she decided to use one of her own remedies. She gave her a teaspoonful of badger fat to swallow and had her wash it down with hot milk. She also had her take some of the fat home and use it on a daily basis. Within a week the troubling cough was gone.* — P. L. / Mundare

## Pneumonia

This is a life-threatening bacterial, viral, or fungal lung inflammation. As the body fights off the infection, the lungs' air sacs fill with thick yellowish green sputum or phlegm, which produces a drowning-like effect. The patient's breathing becomes shallow, rapid, and laboured because of fluid accumulation and reduction of lung capacity.

This serious condition requires medical treatment, and home remedies were limited. Generally, the ill person was kept in bed and well covered with blankets and quilts to induce sweating. Additionally, the following treatments were used:

*Drinking:*
- 1 tbsp., at regular intervals, of wormwood tincture (adult).

*Applying:*
- hot onion poultice to the chest and back (child).
- full-body steam bath, daily, after which the body was well rubbed with a liniment.
- mustard plaster on the chest, reapplied every 4 hours (adult).
- 1 tsp. creosote onto the chest, rubbed in. This was done only for an adult, because it could burn the more sensitive skin of a child.
- cups (wet) or leeches on the chest, followed by a cold compress placed on the back.

## SKIN PROBLEMS

The body's largest organ is also its primary protective barrier against various infections and injuries. When the skin's healthy condition breaks down, this may be expressed as changes in colouration, eruptions, discharges, excessive itchiness, etc. Poor hygiene, limited and primitive sanitary conditions, a restricted diet, and harsh working conditions caused various problems. Working outdoors in all kinds of conditions further stressed skin with the effects of dirt, sweat, sun, and wind. In children, a weaker immune system also led to rashes and other skin irritations.

Many of the problems that developed, such as eczema, boils, and various fungal conditions, were localized and easily treated with home remedies. Some skin rashes were probably evidence of other problems, such as allergies, dry skin, or nutritional deficiencies. These were more difficult to treat.

> To treat skin problems, some people made a fine oil (oliia) by heating sweet cream (solodka smetana) in a pan. The oil that rose to the top of the heated cream was carefully skimmed off and kept in a jar. It was applied to diaper rash, chapped skin, and other skin irritations. — M. P. / Edmonton

The large number and variety of materials used in home treatment suggests that skin problems were common but difficult to treat. Typical home-based treatments involved applying the healing ingredients at least three times a day and ensuring that the area was kept clean, protected, and, if possible, exposed to the sun's healing rays.

Treatments for different skin problems are described below.

## Rashes

*Applying:*
- *Rubbing* on bear fat / **unsalted butter** / fresh cream / pork fat (rancid fat preferred) / lard / oil that accumulates on the top of gently heated sweet cream / human urine / vinegar / baking soda solution / ointments / Vaseline / sulphur added to a zinc-based ointment.
- *Infusion*, washed on or soaked into the problem area 2–3 times daily, of raspberry leaves / nettle leaves / burdock shoots / **wormwood** tops / broad bean leaves / coltsfoot leaves / birchbark.

- *Poultice,* applied and changed 1–2 times daily, of crushed and boiled flax seeds / crushed plantain leaves / yarrow leaves / **coltsfoot** leaves (fuzzy side against the skin) / crushed ground ivy leaves / cactus (aloe) pulp / nettle leaves mixed with salt and egg white.
- *Salve,* applied directly or first placed on brown paper, made from **spruce** *(ialyna)* or pine gum, honey and egg white / mixture (2:1) of sulphur and unsalted butter or rancid pork fat / vegetable oil / sulphur, blue stone (copper sulphate), and lard / **spruce** or pine gum, vegetable oil, sulphur, and young sheep's brain / beef fat, spruce or pine gum, and incense / spruce or pine gum, Vaseline, and egg white / beeswax, lard, spruce or pine gum, and oats / spruce or pine gum and cactus (aloe) pulp / black poplar sap / beeswax, honey, spruce or pine gum, and used axle grease. Most of the salves had the ingredients mixed in equal proportions.
- *Residues:* tar scraped from the inside of a smoking pipe bowl or stem / ash paste from burned white or black poplar wood.
- vegetable oil (hemp and olive were considered the best).
- tobacco leaves that had been soaked overnight in a solution of water and human urine.
- dandelion sap.
- decoction from a whole fireweed plant.

*When someone had a skin condition that would not heal, it was treated with large greenish white, rhubarb-like leaves [coltsfoot?], which were collected from slough edges. The leaves (lystky) were washed, placed white-side-down on the skin, and wrapped on with a cloth. They were left on for a day or two, and then fresh (svizhi) leaves were put on. When the skin started healing, the bandage was removed and the area exposed to the air for more complete healing.* — N. S. / Viking

## Eczema

*Applying:*
- soaking in a decoction of oak bark.
- soil-heated (dark) hemp seed oil (described in chapter nine).

- egg yolk oil (also described in chapter nine).
- salve of spruce or pine gum, unsalted butter, and beeswax.
- mixture, of equal parts, sweet cream and soot from the underside of a stove top plate.
- blue stone (copper sulphate) solution.
- melted beef tallow.

*My husband's younger brother was a cripple (kalika) from birth, and his body became entirely covered with scabs (strupy). His mother had been sick when he was born and another woman had to breastfeed him. People (liudy) said that this was not the right thing to do and that was why he turned out the way he did. A travelling peddler, selling various medicines, suggested that we try an ointment used for horses. My husband's brother used it, and the body rash cleared up completely.* — M. M. / Vegreville

## Impetigo

### Applying:
- salve made of apple tree bark and unsalted butter / goose fat, Vaseline, and kerosene.

*When I was in grade three or four, I caught a skin itch from some kids (dity) in school. They closed the school down for a month and we were given a salve (mast) to treat the itch, but it did not help. We ended up using our own remedy, which was a salve made by mixing rancid pig fat with sulphur. This treatment worked.* — R. B. / Two Hills

## Pimples

### Applying:
- *Poultice* of crushed plantain leaves.
- unsalted butter.

## Cold Sores

### Applying:
- cactus (aloe) pulp or crushed plantain leaves, placed on the sores for 10-15 minutes.
- earwax, put on the sores daily.

## Blisters

### Applying:
- *Poultice* of goose droppings / fresh cow manure.

## Slivers

### Applying:
- *Poultice* of warm milk and bread / moistened homemade soap shavings and sugar.

## Burns

Minor and major burns from fires or hot liquids were a daily household and farm hazard. Children, because of their attraction to, and inexperience with, fire were most vulnerable to being burned. Minimal, temporary damage resulted from first-degree (red and painful area) or second-degree (red, painful, and blistered skin) burns. These were easily and effectively treated with home remedies. Third-degree burns caused more extensive, deeper, more damaging, and permanent injury and often required medical treatment. The most immediate concerns for the first two types of burns, were pain relief and prevention of scarring from the skin drying out and cracking, which could also lead to serious, difficult-to-treat infections. This may be why so many of the home remedies applied an oil or fat to the burn to keep the area soft and moist. This treatment is now recognized as being the wrong thing to do, because fat or oil keep the heat within the skin.

Typical treatments, used daily until healing was complete, included:

*Applying:*

- **goose fat** / unsalted butter / lard (old or rancid pork fat was considered to be the most effective) / lamb fat.
- any vegetable oil (olive, hemp, flax).
- fresh milk / sour milk / **sweet cream** *(solodka smetana)* applied to a cloth and wrapped over the burn.
- finely sieved dry or moistened clay. This was good for preventing scarring in facial burns.
- *Wetting* the burned area with cold water / cold tea / saliva. Salt could be sprinkled on to reduce blistering and speed healing.
- *Salve* made from equal portions of mustard and lard / lard and baking soda / a mixture of young sheep's fat and brain, spruce or pine gum, and vegetable oil / black poplar gum and used axle grease (for severe burns).
- a moist cloth, which was rewet each half hour, wrapped on.
- **Vaseline** or Watkins or Rawleigh **ointments**.
- alcohol, which prevented blistering.
- kerosene.
- vinegar, which relieved pain.
- inner membrane ("skin") of an eggshell, which relieved pain.
- beaten or unbeaten egg white. This was washed off and reapplied regularly. Beating the egg white in homebrew helped prevent infection.
- *Poultice* of crushed **plantain** leaves / coltsfoot leaves / fresh **cow**, horse, or chicken manure, which relieved pain / the slimy algal layer on the surface of a slough or watering trough / coltsfoot leaves / boiled carrots mashed with butter / grated potato / chopped onion / bread soaked in warm milk /
  flour paste.
- rubbing the burned area with the surface of a cut potato / dry or moist baking soda / a piece of soap / aloe vera sap.
- sprinkling puffball spores onto the area, washing them off, and reapplying them. This was done every 8-10 hours to prevent infection.
- melting pig bristles and applying the cooled residue to the burn.

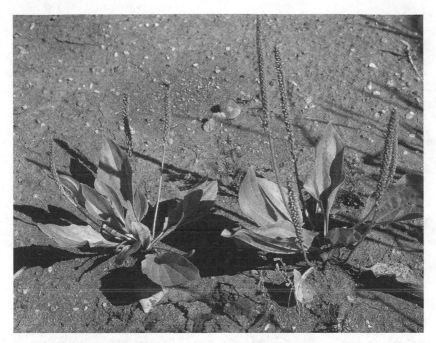

Plantain poultices healed skin conditions very well. [M. MUCZ]

- rabbit skin, placed fur side down on the burned area. This was especially effective on the buttocks and back, where any direct pressure would generate pain and impede healing.

*My two young sons were bathing in a washtub near the stove. When their wash water had cooled, my elder son decided to add some warm water (tepla voda) from a pot on the stove. The water he poured over his younger brother was quite hot and burned his back badly. My son began crying terribly from the pain, and I did not know what to do. My husband's mother was with us, and she quickly went down into our earthen cellar to get some yellow clay (zhovta hlyna). She sifted this on my son's badly burned back and it quickly settled him down. By the next morning the skin was not as red, and after a few more clay treatments it began to heal. I never had to take him to a doctor, and after the skin healed, no scars remained.* — M. P. / Edmonton

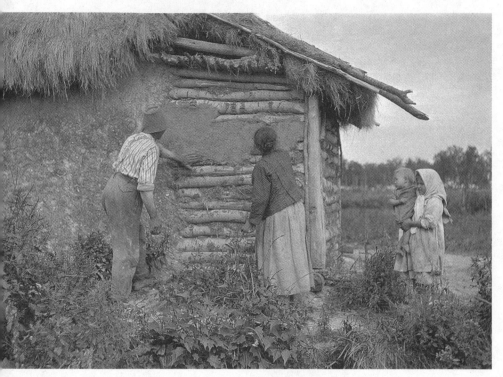

Clay was both a building material and a healing agent. [PAM N9631]

## Frostbite

Frozen or chapped hands and feet were a chronic winter problem for both young and old. These were caused by a lack of adequately warm clothing and appropriate footwear. Exposed skin, as it began to freeze, would initially tingle and eventually become pale and numb as its blood circulation decreased. The proper treatment was to gradually revive the skin was by soaking it in lukewarm water. The worst thing to do, and yet the most common treatment, was to rub the area with snow or ice or place it in cold water. Friction from vigorous rubbing of the limbs may have produced some minor benefit and may have even offset the negative effects of this practice. Fortunately, the majority of frostbite injuries were relatively mild, and in most cases the skin recovered quickly, even with inappropriate treatment.

*We walked* (my ishly) *three miles to school, and in the winter* (vzymku) *we would often get big white patches of frozen skin* (zatyhla shkira) *on our cheeks. We were warned not to put our bare [warm?] hands on these spots because they would leave imprints in the thawed skin. Instead, we were told to pick up snow* (snih) *and rub it on the area.* — C. Z. / Edmonton

Many of the home remedies used were to reduce pain and to prevent the thawed skin from cracking or blistering. These included:

### Applying:

- *Rubbing* on melted sheep fat / unsalted butter / lard / bear grease / sweet cream / oil from heated sweet cream / pig's bile, which was collected when a pig was slaughtered / Vaseline.
- *Soaking* in lanolin-rich water that wool had been washed in / sauerkraut or pickle juice / **kerosene.**
- *Wrapping* on a cloth soaked in kerosene or homebrew.
- *Poultice* of sauerkraut leaves wrapped on and left overnight / coltsfoot leaves / mashed peas. The poultice was changed daily until the skin began to heal.

*My brother froze his feet and hands* (nohy i ruky) *quite badly, but only his fingers* (paltsi) *did not heal and became badly infected. The doctor wanted to cut them all off* (vidrizaty), *but Mother would not agree to this and said she would heal them herself. She had a supply of large dry leaves that had a fuzzy white bottom [coltsfoot?]. She wet these, wrapped them around his fingers, and changed the bandages each morning and evening. She did this for a number of months and saved all his fingers, which he has to this day.* — L. K. / Star

## Warts

Warts are small, hard, round, raised growths on the outer skin. People commonly believed that warts developed from handling frogs and toads, but they are actually growths associated with a viral skin infection. Warts are quite common in children and young adults because of their weaker immune systems. They often appear on the face, fingers, hands, elbows, toes, and soles of the feet, but are more of an inconvenience than a health concern. Even when untreated, they generally disappear on their own, but they can reappear.

> *My uncle had terrible warts* (borodavky) *on his hands, and some Indians gave him a cure for them. He had to cover the warts with his own saliva* (slyna), *but this was only to be done before sunrise and after sunset and never during the day. He did this and they cleared up. He suggested the same treatment for my brother's warts, and they also cleared up in only a week.* — D. A. / Vegreville

Home remedies for warts, which varied from the practical to the supernatural, included:

*Applying:*

- horse sweat or drool / the scrapings of material that accumulates on one's tongue overnight.
- *Wrapping* on a cut clove of garlic / crushed garlic mixed with pork fat / a piece of cut onion, soaked in vinegar for a few hours. These applications were usually left on overnight.
- *Poultice* of crushed or folded plantain leaves / cactus (aloe) pulp / a mustard plaster.
- rubbing the wart with a piece of cut raw potato.
- *Sap* from milkweed / dandelion / sow thistle.
- *Rubbing* on a paste of freshly burned white poplar ashes / homemade laundry soap / used axle grease / school board chalk / rust scraped from old farm machinery.
- *Washing* with blood from a freshly killed pigeon / rinse-water from cleaning sheep's wool / one's own urine.
- *Soaking* in a concentrated salt or stove ash solution.
- *Softening* with water and then scraping off / cutting off the top of the wart, and applying a piece of lye crystal / concentrated iodine /

concentrated nitric acid after the wart was isolated within a circle of Vaseline to prevent damaging healthy skin.

- *Tying off* with a piece of **hair from a horse's tail** / fine silk / linen thread. This was tightened regularly until the wart fell off, which happened in a week or so. The core or "root" could then be pulled or twisted until it came out.
- *Burning* the top off the wart with a hot sewing needle / wire / nail / lit cigarette, and then cutting it off with a sharp razor. This was done regularly until the wart disappeared.

*My brother had bad warts on his hands, and he was told that these were because he had been handling frogs* (zhaby). *Mother knew that the warts could be cured, but only on a certain day of the moon's cycle, which was the full or new moon* (novyi misiats). *The warts had to be washed with the person's own pee on that day and they would then go away. My brother did this, and they disappeared forever. —* L. K. / Star

## Ringworm

This is a common fungal skin infection, in both humans and animals, which develops mainly on the scalp and feet. It is characterized by a crusty ring-like growth that becomes extremely itchy. The condition is highly contagious and can be easily caught from infected cattle, calves, and pigs, as well as from infected humans. Some people believed that it was due to an allergic reaction to certain foods.

Ringworm was treated with a number of home remedies, which included:

### Applying:
- human nasal secretions / earwax / cow urine / fresh cow manure / chicken manure / person's own feces. The smeared area was then wrapped with a clean cloth and changed once or twice daily / residue from the stem of a smoking pipe or burning fresh white or black poplar wood / creoline solution or kerosene. These were strong materials

and produced a burning sensation / egg white / moistened baking soda or sulphur or salt or sugar or powdered copper sulphate or wood ashes / unpasteurized honey.

- *Poultice* of plantain, coltsfoot, or beet leaves.
- *Rubbing* with a salve containing a mixture of pine or spruce gum, vegetable oil, sulphur, and young sheep's fat and brain / sulphur in used axle grease, machinery oil, or animal fat (butter, lard, **goose fat**, or skunk fat) / mashed garlic and stovepipe soot / unsalted butter / Vaseline / used axle grease / used machinery oil.
- *Covering* with a hot cloth compress or a compress soaked in pickle juice / whey.
- *Washing* with rainwater collected from a straw roof (mixed herbal infusion) / liquid from boiled tobacco leaves / wash water from cleaned sheep's wool.
- *Moistening* with heated sour milk / sweet cream / the oily residue developed on gently heated cream.
- letting a puppy lick the area.

*My son had ringworm on his hand, and I was going to take him to a doctor to have it treated. An older man told me that I could treat it myself with a paste of crushed garlic and stove soot* (sazha vid pechi). *This had to be put on the skin infection and then wrapped with a cloth bandage. When I did this, my son began to scream* (krychaty) *from the stinging pain the mixture caused. I quickly washed it off and let it dry. That one short treatment was enough to get rid of the ringworm. — N. H. / Holden*

## Boils

A boil is a painful skin inflammation caused by a bacterial infection of a hair follicle or oil gland. It develops as a reddened swelling with a core of dead tissue surrounded by pus, which forms a whitish to yellowish head. These infections are common on body areas with heavy sweat accumulation, such as the back of the neck, armpits, and groin. They often developed during the busy haying and harvesting seasons when personal hygiene was neglected. Although painful, a boil naturally began to drain in about two weeks and gradually healed within another three to five days.

Boils either were treated intact, which reduced the likilihood of additional infection, or were opened up by pricking the "head" with a heated needle or cutting with a razor. The pus was then squeezed out and the area well cleaned. A better, and less painful, way of opening a boil was to apply a hot pack to the site overnight.

An open and drained boil was washed out with a warm soapy solution or soaked with a hot solution of table salt or Epsom salts (magnesium sulphate). This reduced further inflammation by shrinking the skin tissue and promoted healing. Poultices, the most common follow-up treatment, were usually left on overnight. If they were used during the day, they were changed at least once or twice.

Common home remedies included:

*Applying:*
- *Poultices* made from an **onion** *(tsybulia)* cut in half or crushed, used raw or softened by heating / leaves, entire or mashed, from **coltsfoot** (applied fuzzy side down) / plantain / cow parsnip (wild rhubarb) / geranium / chrysanthemum / cabbage (changed when wilted) / crushed and boiled flax seeds / grated or thinly sliced potatoes / homemade soap and sugar / cow manure / a piece of bread / bread crumbs (heel or crust) soaked in warm fresh or boiled milk and mixed with 1 tbsp. **honey** or sugar / flour dough.
- *Salves and pastes*, often wrapped on with a clean cloth and reapplied 2-3 times daily, made of mustard and lard or badger fat / mustard paste / unsalted butter / stove ashes, soaked in water and made into a paste / dry ashes mixed with vegetable oil / dry ashes rubbed onto the boil / cactus (aloe) sap / softened beeswax / spruce or black poplar gum, heated and strained / baking soda paste / a mixture of equal parts crushed white poplar bark, vegetable oil, sulphur, and sheep fat and brains / a paste made of homemade soap and bread (sometimes chewed up) / a paste made of oily residue from heated fresh cream mixed with flour.
- *Compresses*, applied warm, provided immediate relief and healing by increasing blood flow to the area. They were soaked in plain water / wormwood infusion or decoction / whey.

*A boil* (chyriak) *is best treated by opening it up and draining it. A long-necked (beer or whisky) bottle was held over a steaming kettle to heat the air inside. The opening was placed over the punctured boil and the bottle's heat helped soften the boil. The suction produced by the bottle's air cooling drew the pus out. A hot milk and bread poultice* (pryparka) *was then put on the boil to get it to heal completely.* — J. S. / Lamont

Some less-common treatments included letting a dog, preferably a puppy, lick the boil until it opened up and was cleaned out. The dog's saliva helped in the healing process. Another method was to rub one's own saliva onto the boil. This had to be done every day for a week, before sunrise and after sunset.

*A boil was a terrible thing to get. My daughter and I got them on our necks and they were very painful, but we did not know how to treat them. A neighbour came by and told me of a treatment that the Gypsies* (tsyhany) *used in the Old Country. They would let a dog lick an infected wound or boil until it began healing. We had some pups on the farm, and I took one into my arms, held it to my neck, and let it lick* (lyzaty) *the boils. I did this a number of times, and it did help to clear them up.* — S. R. / Smoky Lake

## Infections

Poor sanitary conditions inside and outside the home, coupled with the need to work even when injured, meant that a minor wound could easily become infected, pus-filled, inflamed, and painful. It was then necessary to open the wound up with a needle sterilized using a match or candle, and to squeeze out the pus. The drained wound was then soaked in hot water (child) or in a hot solution of table salt or Epsom salts (adult) and treated with a home remedy. Extremely infected wounds were soaked in an infusion of wormwood or tansy mustard. Deeply infected wounds were a serious concern, because they could cause blood poisoning. These were taken to a doctor for lancing and treatment with drugs.

*My young brother and I were catching mice* (myshi) *near the haystacks and noticed a larger animal hiding in one of them. My brother, who was the brave one, thought it was only a gopher and quickly reached in to grab it. What he pulled out was a plump rat. His hands were small and he tried to hold onto the rat* (shchur) *by pressing it against his chest. The angry and frightened rat scratched him up badly. The wounds would not heal up, no matter what treatment my mother tried. Even taking him to the doctor did not help. A neighbour suggested putting grated carrots* (tertoi morkvy) *on the infected wounds. The carrot poultice was put on and kept in place with a cloth bandage, and was changed each morning. After only four treatments, the wounds began healing and healed up well.* — P. L. / Mundare

Puffball *(porkhavka)* spores were the most widely used and effective natural antiseptic. Collected when they were ripe (brown and dry), fungal puffballs contained powdery spores that could be applied to infected wounds to promote healing. Home-based treatments for infected wounds were typically reapplied, and dressings changed, once or twice a day. Once healing began, this was then done every two to three days until the wound had healed.

Home treatments varied greatly and consisted of:

### Applying:

Poultices of scalded or crushed leaves from costmary / comfrey / **plantain** / coltsfoot (often moistened with Vaseline, sour milk, sour cream, or sweat from the inner band of a man's hat) / feverfew / horseradish / basil / tobacco / fresh cabbage / lovage / marsh marigold / burdock / cow parsnip (wild rhubarb) / alder (cooked in butter) / split pieces of cactus (aloe) stems or softened pieces of bracket fungus or red top mushroom cap / honey or a honey-and-flour paste / bread dough / grated potato or carrots or beets (sprinkled with sugar) / crushed garlic / chopped, sliced, and heated onions (with or without honey) / crushed, boiled flax seeds / bread soaked in fresh or boiled milk (sometimes with onions or white poplar leaves on top) or sour milk or buttermilk (with plantain leaves on top) / broken pieces of fresh or mouldy bread or bread soaked in milk and honey or sour cream / cattail seeds soaked in milk / flax seeds cooked in milk / moist sugar and homemade soap / clay paste / a moist hot

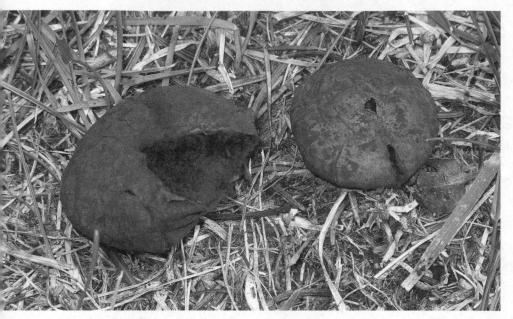

Puffball spores were used as an antiseptic for wounds. [M. MUCZ]

pack / a hot, moist compress / a towel moistened in whitewash (lime) solution.

- *Coating* with a layer of **goose fat** / flax seed oil / skunk fat / rancid unsalted bacon fat / chicken fat / a mixture of rancid unsalted bacon fat, chimney soot, and sulphur / salve made from the fat and brain of a young sheep, spruce or pine gum, and vegetable oil.
- Burning hemp thread on the wound and rubbing the ashes in.
- fresh **cow manure**.
- human urine.
- tincture of Easter lily flowers.

Unusual treatments included:

- letting a puppy lick the wound clean.
- wrapping a piece of baby's placenta, preserved in alcohol, onto the ulcerated wound.

- placing an infected finger inside a hollowed-out pickle and wrapping it on.
- stroking the infected area with a feather to stimulate blood flow to the area.

*I knew a man whose injured leg was not healing, even though it was being treated by a doctor. I told him that I knew a simple cure that would work. He had to go home and urinate* (mochytysia) *on the injured area. He called me crazy but he did try it. The doctor was pleased to see that the wound* (rana) *was healing and believed it was because of the medicine. When told the real remedy, he was not surprised. He said he could also have suggested the same thing, but people would not have thought much of him as a doctor if he did so.* — P. N. / Lamont

## Diaper Rash

Irritated skin on a baby's backside was a common development because diapers were made of cloth (old rags) and were often not changed frequently enough to keep the skin dry. Prolonged contact with urine or feces in the diaper caused the baby's soft, delicate skin to redden and become painfully sore. The rough edges of the diaper often further irritated the area, especially along the thighs. The simplest and most effective home remedy was to bathe the child in a baking soda solution and then to dry the irritated skin gently and thoroughly. Leaving the baby undiapered, and in sunlight, hastened healing.

Additional treatment involved the following:

*Applying:*
- *Rubbing* the area with goose fat / unsalted butter / lard / any available (chicken, duck, etc.) animal fat / vegetable oil such as sunflower, pumpkin seed, hemp, olive / Vaseline.
- *Dusting* with yellow or blue clay that had been crushed and passed through a cheesecloth sieve / flour (burnt or unburnt) / extremely fine (powdery) sand / cornstarch / or puffball spores.
- *Poultice* of fresh wormwood leaves, left on overnight.

## Wounds

Skin abrasions and cuts were daily hazards of farm life, whether during work or play. Sharp field equipment such as axes, scythes, sickles, and saws, and farm tools such as knives and chisels could produce deep and serious wounds. Walking barefoot, a common summer practice of both adults and children, meant additional risk of injury from nails, pegs, sharp stones, twigs, or farm implements. Such accidents produced nasty, dirty puncture wounds that required immediate attention. It was important to first stop the bleeding and then to make certain that the wound was cleaned and protected from infection.

> *When someone had a bleeding wound, they applied "holy mud"* (sviate) *to it. This was made from a mixture of black soil and blessed or holy water* (sviachena voda). *The paste was applied to the wound and kept in place with as cloth bandage.* — N. B. / Edmonton

Puffball mushrooms, valued for their natural antiseptic properties, were collected when they were mature and kept in a paper bag or jar for use throughout the year. Their spores were generally applied to large and deep wounds that could easily become infected, or to already-infected wounds.

In the field, if nothing else was available, the wound was simply tied up with a piece of cloth. Work continued, and the wound was treated later on.

> *When any of us kids got a cut, we simply ran to the field* (pole) *and collected some coltsfoot* (pidbil). *We wrapped it on the wound and continued doing whatever it was we were doing. We always looked after ourselves, because we had a large family* (velyka rodyna) *and could not be always running to Mother for attention.* — C. O. / Edmonton

Different wounds were treated with a wide range of home remedies, and in most cases the same kind of treatment was used on more than one type of wound. These are described below.

### FRESH

Treating these wounds required stopping the bleeding and keeping the affected area clean. The most common treatment was simply to wrap the area tightly with a dry or moistened (cold water) cloth. Bleeding could also be stopped by:

*Applying:*
- crushed yarrow leaves, or pieces of bread from the inner (soft and moist) part of the loaf, wrapped over the wound.
- *Sprinkling* on dry flour / cornstarch / salt / clay / sand / soil / **puffball spores**, or the whole puffball could be applied like a blotter. The wound was then wrapped with a clean cloth.
- softened spruce or pine gum / vinegar.
- ashes from a burned cloth or stove contents.
- juice from crushed yarrow leaves.
- a mat of cobwebs.
- cigarette paper, most often used for small facial nicks produced when shaving
- urinating on the wound, to clean and sterilize it.

*My brother and I were playing on a rail fence* (plit). *I fell off and caught my knee on a nail. It began to bleed badly, and my father carried me quickly into the house. He stopped the bleeding by wrapping on a piece of bread* (shmatok khliba), *from inside the loaf, that had been soaked in milk.* — H. S. / Vegreville

### HEALING

Keeping a wound clean and uninfected helped speed its healing and allowed a protective scab to form. Faster healing also meant less scarring. Healing was promoted by soaking the wound two to three times daily in hot water (child) or in a hot solution of table salt or Epsom salts (adult). If the wound was not healing well, it could be soaked in a hot decoction of speckled alder or young birch branches.

Other treatments included:

*Applying:*
- puffball spores.
- *Botanical poultice* of **plantain** leaves / mashed garlic mixed with goose fat / **coltsfoot** leaves (fuzzy side against the wound) / crushed nettle leaves / crushed or whole birch leaves mixed with bread soaked in milk / crushed lamb's quarters leaves / feverfew leaves / basil leaves / lovage leaves / crushed ground ivy leaves / crushed wild violet leaves / softened bracket fungus / sliced cap of a red top mushroom / grated carrots / grated potatoes / cooked flax seeds / heat-softened sliced onion / fresh cabbage leaf / or cactus (aloe) pulp.
- *Non-botanical poultice* of bread dough / bread soaked in milk or sour cream / slices of softened pig's gallbladder, which had been kept and dried when a pig was slaughtered / chicken fat.
- a paste of vinegar and clay.
- *Rubbing* on iodine / diluted carbolic acid (also used for treating animal wounds) / kerosene / Vaseline / patent ointments / used axle grease.
- *Salves* made from spruce or pine gum, incense, and fresh butter / beeswax, lard, spruce or pine gum, and oats / a mixture of spruce gum and cactus (aloe) pulp.

*Puffball* (porkhavka) *spores were used to stop the bleeding from a bad cut. You kept packing the spores onto the wound* (rana) *and it would soon stop bleeding. Mother had us collect ripe puffballs every fall, and she kept them in a pail* (vidro) *for use on cuts and wounds. I cannot remember a time when she did not have a supply of puffball spores for our family's use.* — M. D. / Vegreville

A simple but effective way of keeping a wound clean and healing was to have a dog lick it on a regular basis. Wounds were also kept clean and soft by applying unsalted butter / goose fat / unsalted lard / sweet cream / badger fat / or honey. These materials helped healing and minimized scar tissue formation.

PUNCTURE

These were serious injuries, because they introduced foreign material into the wound. Initial treatment was similar to that for a shallow injury, where the wound was first soaked in hot water or a hot table salt solution. The difference was that this was done for a longer time (an hour or two) and on a more regular basis (three times a day for three consecutive days). The wound could also be soaked in a wormwood infusion / a decoction of young birch branches / an Epsom salts solution / warm cheese whey / sour milk / kerosene or diluted boric acid. If the puncture wound was shallow, as it often was in a child, it might need only a cleaning with alcohol / iodine / or a dilute carbolic acid solution.

After the initial cleaning, punctures were treated by:

*Applying:*
- *Poultice* of coltsfoot leaves soaked in milk / a bread and sugar mixture / bread soaked in sour milk and covered with plantain leaves / cow manure / heat-softened sliced onions / fresh cabbage leaves / grated potatoes / grated beets / young burdock leaves / plantain leaves / feverfew leaves / lovage leaves / cactus (aloe) pulp / salted pork or unsalted lard

> *My brother's leg was badly cut, down to the bone* (kistka), *and we were unable to get him to the doctor. A female "witch doctor"* (vidma) *lived close to our place, and we had her come over to see what she could do. She looked at the deep wound and told us to cover it with unsalted pork fat* (solonyna). *We wrapped it on the wound and changed it every second day. No infection developed, and the wound healed well.* — M. L. / Vegreville

## Skin Cleanser

Women, with much of their work outdoors, found that their facial skin became dry, toughened, and weathered in appearance. An excellent facial cleanser was made from two tablespoons of finely ground oatmeal and one tablespoon of honey mixed with enough water to make a thin paste. This was applied and left on for fifteen to twenty minutes and then rinsed off with water. It left the skin clean and moist.

> *I had a brown spot on my hand* (ruka) *that was not really sore, but it kept growing. My dad went to my uncle, who was a pipe smoker, and collected some of his pipe ash* (popil vid faiky). *He made a paste with it and applied it to the spot. In a short time the spot disappeared.* — G. T. / Vegreville

# Conclusion ✍

Ukrainian settlers came to Canada materially poor but rich in cultural knowledge and spiritual traditions. Many believed that the opportunity to own a 160-acre homestead in Canada was a divine "gift" to compensate for their poverty and suffering in the Old Country. Little did they know that developing its full potential would require much sweat, toil, and suffering. Their agrarian heritage honoured the soil's life-giving and sustaining potential, so they were more than prepared to pay the price for exacting the riches it offered to those willing to work and persevere.

Elderly grandparents, a common feature of many immigrant families, were a vital resource to not only their children and grandchildren, but to the community at large. They knew from experience how to use the land and its abundant natural resources. Uncertain as to which familiar and useful plants might be found in Canada, many brought their own seeds and cuttings of food and medicinal plant species. Many traditional Ukrainian home-based medicines used plants, such as potatoes, garlic, onions, and cabbage, which were also staple food sources. Native plants with healing applications were the weedy species such as yarrow, coltsfoot, and plantain. These were abundant and widespread through the bloc settlement areas. Knowing that nature can be both friend and foe allowed the settlers to make the most of what was available to them and to protect themselves from the harsh realities of seasonal changes. Natural foods, both plant (berries, mushrooms) and animal (rabbits, game birds, fish), were mainstays of the diet in the early days. Later on, when the homesteads were more self-sufficient, such foods continued to be used as supplements to the regular diet. Wild animal fats, from bears and badgers, became useful healing agents, as did the powdery antiseptic spores of puffball mushrooms.

Limited access to towns and cities meant that self-sufficiency was a necessity of homesteading survival. Doctors and hospitals were uncommon in rural locations, and even if present, their cost was a heavy financial burden that most settlers could ill afford. Similarly, conventional medicines were either costly or not readily available, which meant that inexpensive and available household products and materials became major ingredients of kitchen medicines. Each household depended on the healing capabilities of mothers and, when available, grandmothers, who were the family's main health care providers. Serious health concerns, such as broken bones, pregnancy, and birthing, were entrusted to the community's traditional healers. Bonesetters and midwives served anyone in need and provided highly competent care—even doctors relied on these healers in difficult cases. Persons needing more spiritually based healing sought out the services of a wax pourer, who incorporated faith and prayer into healing. These practitioners dealt with emotionally based issues, such as anxiety, fear, and restlessness—conditions that conventional medicine could not solve.

Homesteaders in the Ukrainian bloc settlements reached out to one another, and each visitor to the home might bring a solution to some existing problem. They shared not only different traditional healing treatments, but also the necessary ingredients. The early homesteaders' survival and success were largely due to their sense of community, which reflected Old Country village traditions and practices.

Recognizing that traditional practices and values prevailed in these ethnically defined settlement areas, city-based specialized traditional healers made regular trips into rural areas to provide services (bloodletting, cupping) and goods (herbal preparations) that Ukrainian immigrants used. Mail-order purchases from catalogues (Eaton's in Winnipeg) made many healing materials (herbs, patent medicines, leeches) accessible for home use. Watkins or Rawleigh salesmen also made regular trips into rural areas and provided a wide range of household products, patent medicines, and much-appreciated medical advice. Various Western newspapers and magazines contained helpful columns, written anonymously by individuals living in similar circumstances, in which applicable household and medical insights were generously shared. Settlers, although geographically isolated, were therefore able to draw on a wide range of resources and knowledge to safely and effectively deal with most of their everyday non-life-threatening health problems. Kitchen medicine was, of necessity, the prevailing form of health care for most homestead families, regardless of their ethnic background.

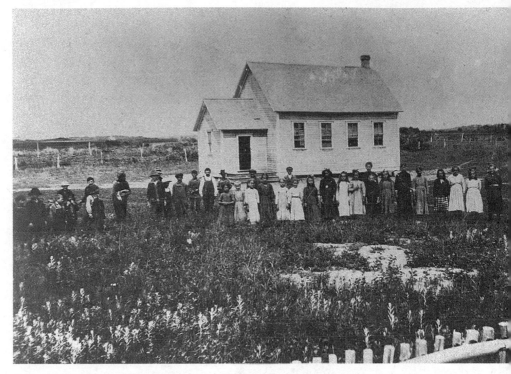

Children, once they were educated in Canadian ways, resisted the use of home remedies. [PAA UV950]

Greater accessibility to and availability of conventional medical resources, such as doctors, pharmacists, dentists, and hospitals, coupled with an increasing ability to pay for such services, greatly transformed rural health care. As the younger generation of Ukrainian Canadians became educated, they became less accepting and tolerant of traditional healing practices. These were often viewed as primitive and backward, suited only to those who were poor and uneducated. Integration into Canadian society required a modernization of lifestyle and health care practices. Folk medicine's potential uses and effectiveness remained, but its application diminished greatly. Many adults of a diverse ethnic backgrounds can readily describe familiar home remedies and treatments. Most kitchen medicine traditions and practices are relegated to stories, shared by grandparents with their grandchildren, about life in the "old days." Sadly, youngsters might question or disbelieve the descriptions of people living in those "old ways."

But the current revival of interest in alternative and holistic medicine suggests that traditional healing knowledge is regaining public favour and support. Home remedies could, and should, be more widely used in the treatment of simple everyday health problems such as cuts, scrapes, headaches, and sniffles. Application of kitchen medicine practices would empower people to understand their capacity to heal themselves with simple, commonly available resources. This would substantially free conventional medicine to focus its time and finances on more serious and critical health issues, such as cancer, diabetes, and heart disease. These and other life-threatening illnesses require sophisticated technological intervention for effective treatment.

Such a dichotomy of treatments—traditional as well as conventional—would unite traditional folk medicine's roots with the fruits of advanced scientific medical knowledge and practices. We could once again recognize that Mother Nature provides us with innumerable resources to not only heal ourselves, but also to stay healthy. Society would benefit greatly if kitchen medicine, practised and refined by our ancestors, once again became a part of daily life. Such a development would bring our lives into greater balance and harmony with nature. I hope that the knowledge contained in this book can act as a bridge between the past and the future. The simplicity and integrity of kitchen medicine has no boundaries in time and space, other than our willingness to know, understand, and accept its potential to serve humanity as it once did.

## Personal history and ethnobotanical questions asked of the informants during audiotaped interviews

### PERSONAL HISTORY

Informant's name / maiden name
Current address
Birth: date / place
Settlement area: initial / permanent
Education
Religious affiliation
Marriage: date / spouse's name (birth date / birthplace / religion)
Family size: daughters / sons
Parents: names / origins / number of children

### ETHNOBOTANICAL INFORMATION

Homestead vegetation resources
Building and tool construction materials
Household items
Heating fuel

Crafts and ornaments
Plant-based dyes
Textiles

Home remedies: conditions treated / materials and preparation / veterinary applications
Remedies obtained from other peoples: Native / other ethnic groups
Community-based healers: herbalists / midwives / bonesetters / wax pourers

Plant-based foods
Plants grown: house / garden
Garden features
Animal feed

Personal hygiene
Religious practices and superstitions

## English, scientific, and Ukrainian names for native fungal and plant species used in home remedies

| English name | Scientific name* | Ukrainian name |
|---|---|---|
| *Fungi:* | | |
| birch polypore | *Piptoporus betulinus* | hirkyi hryb |
| chaga / birch canker | *Inonotus obliquus* | berezovyi hryb |
| common puffball | *Lycoperdon perlatum* | porkhavka |
| giant puffball | *Calvatia cyathiformis* | porkhavka |
| *Spore-bearing plants:* | | |
| common horsetail | *Equisetum arvense* | sosonka / khovoshch |
| fern | species unidentified | paporot |
| *Grasses:* | | |
| cattail | *Typha latifolia* | rohiz |
| couch grass | *Elymus repens* | pyrii |
| *Broad-leaved plants:* | | |
| cow parsnip | *Heracleum maximum* | borshchivnyk |
| lily of the valley | *Maianthemum canadense* | vesnivka |
| arrow-leaved coltsfoot | *Petasites sagittatus* | pidbil / pidlibuk / kremena / babka** |
| Seneca root | *Polygala senega* | kytiaky |
| strawberry | *Fragaria spp.* | sunytsi / iahody |
| three-flowered avens | *Geum triflorum* | hravilat |
| violet | *Viola spp.* | fialka |

| English name | Scientific name* | Ukrainian name |
| --- | --- | --- |
| *Weeds:* | | |
| black henbane | *Hyoscamus niger* | blekota |
| broad-leaved plantain | *Plantago major* | podorozhnyk / babka** |
| Canada thistle | *Cirsium arvense* | osot |
| common burdock | *Arctium minus* | lopukh |
| common dandelion | *Taraxacum officinale* | kulbaba |
| common mullein | *Verbascum thapsus* | dyvyna |
| common tansy | *Tanacetum vulgare* | pyzhmo / kanfrii |
| dock | *Rumex spp.* | shchavel / kvasok |
| lamb's quarters | *Chenopodium album* | loboda / natyna |
| pineapple weed | *Matricaria matricarioides* | romashka |
| sow thistle | *Sonchus spp.* | molochak |
| stinging nettle | *Urtica diocia* | kropyva |
| wormwood / absinth | *Artemisia absinthium* | polyn |
| yarrow | *Achillea millefolium* | derevii / krivavnyk |
| *Shrubs:* | | |
| blueberry | *Vaccinium myrtilloides* | chornytsia |
| chokecherry | *Prunus virginiana* | cheremkhy |
| common bearberry | *Arctostaphylos uva-ursi* | muchnytsia |
| creeping juniper | *Juniperus horizontalis* | ialovets |
| currant | *Ribes spp.* | porichky |
| highbush cranberry | *Viburnum trilobum* | kalyna |
| lowbush cranberry | *Viburnum edule* | kalyna |
| pin cherry | *Prunus pennsylvanica* | cheremkhy |
| raspberry | *Rubus spp.* | malyna / malyny |
| rose | *Rosa spp.* | shypshyna / rozha / dyka ruzha |
| round-leaved hawthorn | *Crataegus chrysocarpa* | hlid |
| willow | *Salix spp.* | verba / loza |
| *Trees:* | | |
| balsam poplar | *Populus balsamifera* | topolia |
| linden | *Tilia spp.* | lypa |
| oak | *Quercus spp.* | dub |
| paper birch | *Betula papyrifera* | bereza |

| English name | Scientific name* | Ukrainian name |
|---|---|---|
| pine | *Pinus spp.* | sosna |
| spruce | *Picea spp.* | ialyna / smereka |
| speckled alder | *Alnus incana* | vilkha |
| trembling aspen | *Populus tremuloides* | osyka / topolia / trepeta |

\* Only a genus name is provided when a specific species was not identified by informants.
\*\* The term *babka* was widely applied to any important and widely used healing plant.

## English, scientific, and Ukrainian names for domesticated garden plants used in home remedies

| English name | Scientific name | Ukrainian name |
| --- | --- | --- |
| aloe | *Aloe vera* | aloe |
| asparagus | *Asparagus officinalis* | kholodok |
| bachelor button | *Centaurea cyanus* | voloshka |
| basil | *Ocimum basilicum* | bazylik |
| bean | *Phaseolus vulgaris* | kvasolia / fasolia |
| beet | *Beta vulgaris* | buriak |
| cabbage | *Brassica oleracea* | kapusta |
| caraway | *Carum carvi* | kmyn |
| carrot | *Daucus carota* | morkva |
| celery | *Apium graveolens* | selera |
| chamomile | *Matricaria chamomilla* | romashka / rum'ianka / romanets |
| comfrey | *Symphytum officinale* | zhyvokist |
| costmary | *Chrysanthemum balsamita* | kanuper |
| dill | *Anethum graveolens* | krip |
| fern | species unknown | paporot |
| feverfew | *Tanacetum parthenium* | maruna / marunka |
| garlic | *Allium sativum* | chasnyk |
| horseradish | *Armoracia rusticana* | khrin |
| lovage | *Levisticum officinale* | liubystok |

| English name | Scientific name | Ukrainian name |
| --- | --- | --- |
| marigold | *Calendula officinalis* | nahidky / chornobryvtsi |
| mint | *Mentha spp.* | m'iata / mietka |
| onion | *Allium cepa* | tsybulia |
| opium poppy | *Papaver somniferum* | mak |
| parsley | *Petroselinum crispum* | petrushka |
| parsnip | *Pastinaca sativa* | pasternak / postyrnak |
| pea | *Pisum sativum* | horokh |
| potato | *Solanum tuberosum* | kartoplia / barabolia |
| radish | *Raphanus sativus* | redka / redyska |
| rhubarb | *Rheum spp.* | revin |
| sage | *Salvia officinalis* | shavliia |
| thyme | *Thymus vulgaris* | chybryk |
| tobacco | *Nicotiana tabacum* | tiutiun |
| turnip | *Brassica rapa* | ripa |
| sweet william | *Dianthus barbatus* | kashtanchyky / hvozdyky |

## English, scientific, and Ukrainian names for domesticated crop plants used in home remedies

| English name | Scientific name | Ukrainian name |
| --- | --- | --- |
| alfalfa | *Medicago sativa* | liutserna |
| barley | *Hordeum vulgare* | iachmin |
| buckwheat | *Fagopyrum esculentum* | hrechka |
| clover | *Trifolium spp.* | koniushyna |
| flax | *Linum usitatissimum* | lon |
| hemp | *Cannabis sativa* | konopli / kanopli |
| oats | *Avena sativa* | oves |
| rye | *Secale cereale* | zhyto |

## Modified Library of Congress (MLC) transliterations of the Ukrainian alphabet into the English alphabet, for terms and phrases used in the text

| Ukrainian | MLC | "Sound" | Ukrainian | MLC | "Sound" |
|-----------|-----|---------|-----------|-----|---------|
| А | a | ah | Н | n | en |
| Б | b | beh | О | o | oh |
| В | v | veh | П | p | peh |
| Г | h | heh | Р | r | err |
| Ґ | g | geh | С | s | ess |
| Д | d | deh | Т | t | teh |
| Е | e | eh | У | u | oo |
| Є | ie | yeh | Ф | f | ef |
| Ж | zh | zheh | Х | kh | khah |
| З | z | zeh | Ц | ts | tseh |
| И | y | ih | Ч | ch | cheh |
| І | i | ee | Ш | sh | shah |
| Ї | i | yee | Щ | shch | shchah |
| Й | i | yot | Ю | iu | yoo |
| К | k | kah | Я | ia | yah |
| Л | l | el | Ь | ' | (soft sign) |
| М | m | em | | | |

# Selected Readings ✑

Alberta Rose Historical Society. *Pride in Progress: Chipman, St. Michael, Star, and Districts*. Chipman, AB: Alberta Rose Historical Society, 1983.

Andrew Historical Society. *Dreams and Destinies: Andrew and District*. Andrew, AB: Andrew Historical Society, 1980.

Balan, J. *Salt and Braided Bread: Ukrainian Life in Canada*. Toronto: Oxford University Press, 1984.

Borowsky, M.L. *Plants from Ukraine in Canada*. Winnipeg: Ukrainian Free Academy of Sciences, 1975.

Bruderheim Historical Committee. *From Bush to Bushels: A History of Bruderheim and District*. Bruderheim, AB: Bruderheim Historical Committee, 1983.

Burke, M.V. *The Ukrainian Canadians*. Toronto: Van Nostrand Reinhold Ltd., 1978.

Champ, J. "Pioneer cure-alls: The use of home remedies and patent medicines in rural Saskatchewan, 1900–1930." Saskatoon: Western Development Museum Curatorial Centre, 2001.

Charuk, M., ed. *The History of Willingdon: 1928–1978*. St. Paul, AB: L.H. Drouvin, St. Paul Journal, 1978.

Czumar, W.A. *Recollections About the Life of the First Ukrainian Settlers in Canada*. Edmonton: Canadian Institute of Ukrainian Studies, 1981.

Doroshenko, D. *A Survey of Ukrainian History*. Edited and updated by O.W. Gerus. Winnipeg: Trident Press, 1984.

Drouin, L. *History of St. Paul, 1909–1959*. St. Paul, AB: St. Paul Journal, 1960.

Dziadyk, A. *Smiles and Tears: About Our Pioneers*. Saskatoon: Prairie Gold Publishing, 2005.

Ewach, H. *The Call of the Land: A Short Story of Life in Canada*. Winnipeg: Trident Press, 1986.

Ewanchuk, M. *Spruce, Swamp, and Stone: History of the Pioneer Ukrainian Settlement in the Gimli Area*. Steinbach, MB: Derksen Printers, 1977.

——. *Pioneer Profiles: Ukrainian Settlers in Manitoba*. Steinbach, MB: Derksen Printers, 1981.

——. *Pioneer Settlers: Ukrainians in the Dauphin Area 1896–1926*. Steinbach, MB: Derksen Printers, 1988.

——. *Reflections and Reminiscences: Ukrainians in Canada 1892–1992*. Steinbach, MB: Derksen Printers, 1995.

——. *East of the Red: Early Ukrainian Settlements, 1896–1930*, vol. 1. Steinbach, MB: Derksen Printers, 1998.

——. *East of the Red: Early Ukrainian Settlements North of the Dawson Trail*, vol. 2. Steinbach, MB: Derksen Printers, 1999.

——. *Growing Up on a Bush Homestead: Pioneer Life as Seen From the Eyes of Children*. Steinbach, MB: Derksen Printers, 2003.

Gerus, O.W., and J.E. Rea. *The Ukrainians in Canada*. Ottawa: Canadian Historical Association, Booklet no. 10, 1985.

Glebe, H.J., ed. *Pulse to Pen: Remembering When; A Collection of True Stories by Prairie Pioneers*. Winnipeg: Hignell Printing, 1992.

Goa, D., ed. *The Ukrainian Religious Experience: Tradition and the Canadian Cultural Context*. Edmonton: Canadian Institute of Ukrainian Studies Press, 1989.

Hanchuk, R.J. *The Word and Wax: A Medical Folk Ritual Among Ukrainians in Alberta*. Canadian Series in Ukrainian Ethnology, vol. 2. Edmonton: Canadian Institute of Ukrainian Studies Press, 1999.

Harbuz, M. *Ukrainian Pioneer Days in Early Years 1898–1916 in Alvena and District, Saskatchewan*. North Battleford, SK: Appel Printing, 1980.

Himka, J.P. *Galicia and Bukovina*. Edmonton: Alberta Culture and Multiculturalism, Historic Sites Service (Occasional Paper no. 20), 1990.

Hrushevsky, M. *A History of Ukraine*. New Haven, CT: Yale University Press, 1941.

Hrynchuk, A., and J. Klufas, eds. *Memories: Redwater and District*. Calgary: D.W. Friesen, 1972.

Hryniuk, L. *Canada's Ukrainians*. Toronto: University of Toronto Press, 1991.

Humeniuk, P. *Hardship and Progress of Ukrainian Pioneers: Memoirs from Stuartborn Colony and Other Points*. Steinbach, MB: Derksen Printers, 1975.

Kaye, V.J. *Early Ukrainian Settlements in Canada 1895–1900: Dr. Josef Oleskow's Role in the Settlement of the Canadian Northwest*. Toronto: University of Toronto Press, 1964.

Keywan, Z., and M. Coles. *Greater Than Kings: Ukrainian Pioneer Settlement in Canada*. Montreal: Harvest House, 1977.

Klymasz, A.K. "Folk Medicine: A Ukrainian Canadian Experience." Master of Arts thesis. Winnipeg: Department of Anthropology, University of Manitoba, 1991.

Klymasz, R. *The Ukrainians in Canada 1891–1991*. Hull, QC: Canadian Museum of Civilization, 1991.

——. In R.B. Bilash, ed. *Sviéto: Celebrating Ukrainian-Canadian Ritual in East Central Alberta Through the Generations*. Edmonton: Alberta Culture and Multiculturalism, Historic Sites and Archives Service (Occasional Paper no. 21), 1992.

Knab, S.H. *Polish Herbs, Flowers & Folk Medicine*. New York: Hippocrene Books, 1995.

Kostash, M. *All of Baba's Children*. Edmonton: Hurtig, 1977.

Kourennoff, P.M. *Russian Folk Medicine*. Translated and edited by G. St. George. London: Pan Books, 1970.

Kubijovyc, V. *Encyclopedia of Ukraine*. Toronto: University of Toronto Press, 1988.

Kuropas, M.B. *The Ukrainian Americans: Roots and Aspirations 1884–1954*. Toronto: University of Toronto Press, 1991.

Lazarenko, J.M., ed. *The Ukrainian Pioneers in Alberta*. Edmonton. Ukrainian Pioneers' Association of Alberta, 1970.

Lehr, J. *Ukrainian Vernacular Architecture in Alberta*. Edmonton: Alberta Culture and Multiculturalism, Historic Sites and Archives Service (Occasional Paper no. 1), 1976.

——. *Homesteading on the Prairies: Iwan Mihaychuk*. Toronto: Heritage Series, 1990.

Lesoway, M. *Out of the Peasant Mold: A Structural History of the M. Hwareliak Home in Shandro, Alberta*. Edmonton: Alberta Culture and Multiculturalism, Historical Resources Division (Occasional Paper no. 16), 1989.

Lewis, N.L. "Goose Grease and Turpentine: Mother Treats the Family's Illnesses." *Prairie Forum* 15, no. 1 (1990): 67–84.

Luciuk, L., and S. Hryniuk, eds. *Canada's Ukrainians: Negotiating an Identity*. Toronto: Ukrainian Canadian Centennial Committee and University of Toronto Press, 1991.

Lupul, M.R., ed. *A Heritage in Transition: Essays in the History of Ukrainians in Canada*. Toronto: McClelland & Stewart, 1982.

——. *Visible Symbols: Cultural Expression Among Canada's Ukrainians*. Edmonton: Canadian Institute of Ukrainian Studies Press, 1984.

——. *Continuity and Change: The Cultural Life of Alberta's First Ukrainians*. Edmonton: Canadian Institute of Ukrainian Studies Press, 1988.

Lysenko, V. *Men in Sheepskin Coats: A Study in Assimilation*. Toronto: Ryerson Press, 1947.

MacGregor, J.G. *Vilni Zemli (Free Lands): The Ukrainian Settlement of Alberta*. Toronto: McClelland & Stewart, 1969.

Magocsi, P.R. *Ukraine: A Historical Atlas*. Toronto: University of Toronto Press, 1985.

Martynowych, O.T. *The Ukrainian Bloc Settlement in East Central Alberta, 1890–1930: A History*. Edmonton: Historic Sites and Archives Service (Occasional Paper no. 10), Alberta Culture and Multiculturalism, 1985.

——. *Ukrainians in Canada: The Formative Years, 1891–1924*. Edmonton: Canadian Institute of Ukrainian Studies Press, 1991.

Marunchak, M.H. *The Ukrainian Canadians: A History*. Winnipeg: Ukrainian Free Academy of Sciences, 1970.

Melnycky, P. *Shelter, Feed and Dray: A Structural History of the Radway Livery Barn*. Edmonton: Alberta Culture and Multiculturalism, Historical Resources Division (Occasional Paper no. 18), 1988.

Momryk, M. *A Guide to Sources for the Study of Ukrainian Canadians: National Ethnic Archives*. Ottawa: Ethnic Archives of Canada, 1984.

Moore, J. *The Saskatchewan Secret: Folk Healers, Diviners, and Mystics of the Prairies*. Regina: Benchmark Press, 2010.

Mundare Historical Society. *Memories of Mundare: A History of Mundare and Districts*. Mundare, AB: Mundare Historical Society, 1980.

Myroniuk, H. *Ukrainians in North America: A Selected Bibliography*. St. Paul, MN: Immigration History Research Center, University of Minnesota, 1981.

Nahachewsky, A. *Ukrainian Dug-out Dwellings in East Central Alberta*. Edmonton: Alberta Culture and Multiculturalism, Historic Sites Service (Occasional Paper no. 11), 1985.

Nay, M.A. *Trailblazers of Ukrainian Emigration to Canada: Wasyl Eleniuk and Ivan Pylypow*. Edmonton: Brightest Pebble Publishing, 1997.

Osadcha-Janata, N. *Herbs Used in Ukrainian Folk Medicine*. New York: New York Botanical Garden, 1952.

——. *Ukrains'ki narodni nazvy roslyn* [Plant Names in Ukrainian Vernacular]. New York: Ukrainian Academy of Arts and Sciences in the United States, 1973.

Paximadis, M. *Look Who's Coming: The Wachna Story*. Oshawa, ON: Miracle Press, 1976.

Petryshyn, J. *Peasants in a Promised Land: Canada and the Ukrainians, 1891–1914*. Toronto: James Lorimer & Company, 1985.

Pinuita, H. "The Organizational Life of Ukrainian Canadians." Master of Arts thesis. Ottawa: University of Ottawa, 1952.

——. *Land of Pain, Land of Promise: First Person Accounts by Ukrainian Pioneers 1891–1914*. Saskatoon: Western Producer Prairie Books, 1978.

Potrebenko, H. *No Streets of Gold: A Social History of Ukrainians in Alberta*. Vancouver: New Star Books, 1977.

Ranfurly History Book. *Memories of Ranfurly Pioneer Years: A History of Avon, Birch Hill, Hamburg, Hillock and Lampburg School Districts*. Ranfurly, AB: Ranfurly History Book, 1983.

Rollings-Magnusson, S. "Flax Seed, Goose Grease, and Gun Powder: Medical Practices By Women Homesteaders in Saskatchewan (1882–1914)." *Journal of Family History* 33, no. 4 (2008): 388–410.

Romaniuk, G. *Taking Root in Canada: An Autobiography*. Winnipeg: Columbia Press, 1954.

Rozumnyj, J., ed. *New Soil, Old Roots: The Ukrainian Experience in Canada*. Winnipeg: Ukrainian
    Academy of Arts and Sciences in Canada, 1983.

Skwarok, J. *The Ukrainian Settlers in Canada and Their Schools, 1891–1921*. Edmonton: Basilian Press, 1958.

Smoky Lake and District Cultural and Heritage Society. *Our Legacy: History of Smoky Lake and Area*.
    Smoky Lake, AB: Smoky Lake and District Cultural and Heritage Society, 1983.

Stainton, I.H., and E.C. Carlsson, eds. *Lamont and District: Along Victoria Trail*. Lamont, AB: Lamont and
    District Historian, 1978.

Stechishin, J.V. *A History of Ukrainian Settlement in Canada*. Winnipeg: Trident Press, 1992.

Subtelny, O. *Ukrainians in North America: An Illustrated History*. Toronto: University of Toronto Press, 1991.

Tesarski, F. *Son of Pioneers*. Winnipeg: Hignell Printing, 1987.

Tomyn, M.H. *A Treasury of Historic Snippets: Town and Country*. Edmonton: Arrow Media, 1994.

Two Hills Historical Society. *Down Memory Trails: A History of Two Hills and Surrounding Area*. Two Hills,
    AB: Two Hills Historical Society, 1986.

Ukrainian Pioneers' Association of Alberta. *Ukrainians in Alberta*. Edmonton: Ukrainian Pioneers'
    Association of Alberta, 1975.

——. *Ukrainians in Alberta*, vol. 2. Winnipeg: Trident Press, 1981.

Vegreville and District Historical Society. *Vegreville in Review: History of Vegreville and Surrounding Area,
    1880–1980*. (2 vols.) Vegreville, AB: Vegreville and District Historical Society, 1980.

Woycenko, O. *The Ukrainians in Canada* (2nd ed.). Winnipeg: Trident Press, 1968.

Yopik, H.A. *Ukrainian Canadian Archives and Museum of Alberta: Artifacts of Ukrainian Pioneers of Alberta*.
    Edmonton: Ukrainian Canadian Archives and Museum of Alberta Publication no. 11, 1987.

Young, C.H. *The Ukrainian Canadians: A Study in Assimilation*. Toronto: Thomas Nelson & Sons, 1931.

Yuzyk, P. *The Ukrainians in Manitoba: A Social History*. Toronto: University of Toronto Press, 1953.

——. *Ukrainian Canadians*. Toronto: Ukrainian Canadian Business and Professional Federation, 1967.

Zazula, W. *Pioneer Memories: Reminiscences*. Edmonton: Alpha-One Printers, 1983.

Zevin, I.V., N. Altman, and L.V. Zevin. *A Russian Herbal: Traditional Remedies for Health and Healing*.
    Rochester, NY: Healing Arts Press, 1997.

## Dictionaries Used for Ukrainian Transliteration

Andrusyshen, C.H. *Ukrainian-English Dictionary*. Toronto: University of Toronto Press, 1993.

Niniows'kyi, W. *Ukrainian-English and English-Ukrainian Dictionary* (2nd ed.) Edmonton: Ukrainian
    Bookstore, 1990.

# Index ✍

Page numbers in *italics* refer to photographs.
A page number with a *t* refers to a table.

manipulation-based healing practices, 77–78, 79t

manure treatments
    crippled feet, 134
    infections, 28, 39, 57, 59, 156, 192, 222
    puncture wounds, 28, 227
    in remedies, 57, 58t, 59
    skin problems, 211, 212, 217

mare's milk, 58t

marigold (nahidky / chornobryvtsi), 221

maruna / marunka. See feverfew

massage, 77, 79t, 86, 122–25

measles
    farm materials as remedies, 58t
    manipulation- or application-based
        remedies, 77, 79t
    overview of, 150
    variety of remedies, 43, 44t

med. See honey

medical doctors and hospitals
    broken bones, 132
    childbirth, 23, 163–64
    costs and payment systems, 25, 27, 30, 230
    druggists, 30, 106
    folk medicine and, 19–20, 21, 27–28, 121,
        223, 230
    history of, 11–12
    hospitals, 15, 27, 29, 230
    naturopathic doctors, 25, 50
    overview of, 27–30
    scarcity of, 15, 27
    suspicion of, 15, 28, 45
    See also dental problems

medicinal whisky. See homebrew; whisky

medicine man or woman. See spiritual healers
    and healing

menstruation
    "bad" blood in menopause, 81
    manipulation- or application-based
        remedies, 80t
    overview of, 158–59
    patent medicines, 73t
    plant-based remedies, 53t, 66t, 71t
    variety of remedies, 44t

midwives
    overview of, 22–24, 162–64
    treatments by, 44, 100

See also birth control and abortion;
    childbirth; pregnancy

milk
    cold and flu remedies, 143, 205
    gastrointestinal remedies, 178, 196
    with opium poppy extracts, 146
    in poultices, 109, 220, 225
    in remedies, 57, 58t
    sore throat remedies, 186, 188
    tuberculosis remedy, 148

minerals and vitamins from tonics, 116

mint (m'iata / mietka), 69, 70t, 73t

mites, 200

molasses, 53t

monkshood, 71t

moonshine. See homebrew

morning sickness, 163

mothers
    as healers, 16, 17, 49
    large families, 22, 161, 164

moulds as remedies, 68

mullein, 66t

mumps, 32, 43

musculoskeletal problems
    types treated, 38t, 39
    variety of remedies, 42t, 43
    See also abdominal strain; aches and pains;
        arthritis and rheumatism; breaks and
        sprains; chilled body; foot and hand
        problems

mustard
    plasters, 110–11, 125, 187, 203
    in remedies, 53t, 54, 176

narcotics. See poppy, opium

nasal congestion, 204–05
    See also congestion, respiratory

Native healing. See Aboriginal healing
    traditions

naturopathic doctors, 25, 50

nervousness. See emotional problems

nettle, stinging (kropyva)
    for arthritis, 62, 65, 131, 132, 133
    in remedies, 66t, 165

newborns. See infants and newborns

nitric acid, 56t

# Other Titles from The University of Alberta Press

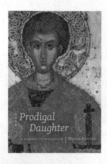

Prodigal Daughter
*A Journey to Byzantium*
MYRNA KOSTASH
352 pages | Map, bibliography, index
Wayfarer Series
978-0-88864-534-0 | $34.95 (T) paper
Travel Memoir/Creative Nonfiction

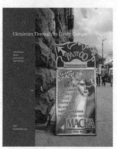

Ukrainian Through its Living Culture
*Advanced Level Language Textbook*
ALLA NEDASHKIVSKA
368 pages | Full-colour throughout, illustrations,
photographs, subject index, glossary
978-0-88864-517-3 | $60.00 (X) cloth
Ukrainian Language/Linguistics

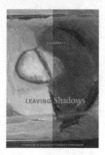

Leaving Shadows
*Literature in English by Canada's Ukrainians*
LISA GREKUL
296 pages | Introduction, notes, bibliography, index
A volume in cuRRents, a Canadian literature series
978-0-88864-452-7 | $34.95 (S) paper
Literary Criticism/Canadian Literature